LIFEBEATS

Linda Strangio, RN, MA, CCRN

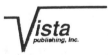

Vista
publishing, Inc.

Copyright © 1996 by Linda Strangio

Edited by Carolyn S. Zagury, MS, RN, CPC

Cover Design by Thomas Taylor of Thomcatt Graphics

Vista Publishing, Inc.
473 Broadway
Long Branch, NJ 07740
(908) 229-6500

This publication is written for the reading pleasure of the general public. The author is solely responsible for the content of the written work and has fictionalized the stories, characters and places in this publication in order to protect any issues of confidentiality.

Printed and bound in the United States of America

First Edition

ISBN: 1-880254-39-5

Library of Congress Catalog Card Number: 96-60791

U.S.A. Price $12.95
Canada Price $17.95

DEDICATION

I dedicate *Lifebeats* to the Department of Radiology of The Mountainside Hospital, Montclair, New Jersey.

- - - To the staffs of C.T. Scanning, Diagnostic X-Ray, M.R.I., Nuclear Medicine, Special Procedures, and Ultrasound.

- - - To the radiological technologists who consistently treat all patients with caring, compassion, and dignity, and whose expertise is surpassed by none.

- - - To the radiologists whose skills and abilities result in the highest quality of patient care, and who treat the radiology nurses as colleagues.

- - - To the other radiology nurses, my wonderful partners.

- - - To the radiology support staff without whom there would be no department.

I consider myself privileged to be a part of this very special group.

I also dedicate this book to my forever family of Mountainside's Surgical I.C.U.

And again, to my mother. LOOK, MA, I DID IT AGAIN !!!

SPECIAL THANKS

--- To the staffs of *Nursing Spectrum* who supported and encouraged me, and who printed some of my stories and then released them to me so that I could use them in this book.

--- To Carol Larkin R.N., my clone, who sang the praises of *To Be A Nurse*, and who kept me motivated to write *Lifebeats* by constantly saying, "Read me another story!"

--- To Kathy Williams R.N. and Sally Starin R.N., who became my unofficial agents for *To Be A Nurse*, and cheered me on for this book.

--- To the staff of The Mountainside Hospital, for continuously making me feel like a celebrity.

--- To my husband, Vinny, who helped me out with my many computer questions.

--- And to Carol Zagury, who kept my dream alive.

THANK YOU, ALL OF YOU. WITHOUT YOU, THERE WOULD BE NO

LIFEBEATS!

MEET THE AUTHOR

Linda Strangio has an identical twin sister, who is also a nurse. Born in Brooklyn, they both graduated from the Mount Sinai Hospital School of Nursing in New York City and continue to practice full time hospital nursing.

Besides holding national certification in critical care nursing (C.C.R.N.), Linda also has two degrees in psychology. She has written for many national and tri-state magazines and journals, and her first book, *To Be A Nurse*, was released last year. She is a member of nine professional organizations.

Linda's experience covers many years in critical care nursing, where she has been a staff nurse, head nurse, and patient care coordinator. For the past four years, she has been the radiology nursing coordinator for the department of radiology at The Mountainside Hospital, Montclair, New Jersey.

She has been married for twenty-nine years and has three grown children. Linda lives with her husband in New Jersey, where she spends much of her free time writing and crocheting.

TABLE OF CONTENTS

INTRODUCTION

Lifebeats.

As the heart pumps its precious fluid to nourish the body, life itself sends us what we need to feed the soul. And there is with happiness and joy as well as sorrow and grief.

Nursing, perhaps more than any of the helping professions, gives us the opportunity to be part of people's lives. This book is an accumulation of the different beats, the happy ones as well the sad, and portrays life through the eyes of a nurse.

Lifebeats is a collection of true stories based on real people. The names and events, though changed to protect privacy and confidentiality, reflect the truth. The stories come from a variety of sources, and no particular hospital or health care facility is described. Some are compilations of experiences, but all of them really happened.

Some of these stories will make the reader smile, while others may bring a tear. But they are all a part of our living and dying and loving and laughing. And that's what life is all about.

Lifebeats.

Prologue

After my last book, *To Be A Nurse*, was published, people started to ask me when I was going to write the sequel. Never, I told them. How could there be a sequel? *To Be A Nurse* was made of seventy-four stories, and that was the end of it. After all, how could there be more than seventy-four stories about what it means to be a nurse?

Well, how very wrong I was! This book, *Lifebeats*, has sixty-four stories, all new and all different. As I wrote some of them, the memories made me smile, and at times I even laughed out loud. With others, I found myself tense and angry, and once in a while, on the verge of tears. As I wrote, something made me think of something else. And before I knew it, there was my next story.

I used to wonder how the cast of a long playing Broadway show could keep fresh and enthusiastic every day. How on earth could they do the same thing over and over again, seven days a week? Why, they must simply go through the motions, I thought. But as I began to write these stories, I found the answer. The audience is different. Every day and every performance. That keeps them going. And patients are the nurse's audience and the hospital, or wherever he or she practices, is the theater.

Just as the audience changes for the cast, so do the patients for the nurse. The lady who had a bowel resection last week and was in room 621 is not the same as the lady in that bed today who has undergone the same operation. Patients are people and every person is a distinct and very different human being, with special needs and unique circumstances.

People ask me questions like, "Did you ever hear of such and such?" Or "Did you ever see this or that?" Yes. I've seen it all and I've done it all. I've been there. Over and over again. And it never gets boring.

And that's why there will always be stories. As long as there are people who laugh and cry and hurt and need, there will be nurses who have been privileged to become part of their sorrows and their joys. To be a nurse is like nothing else. It makes us one with the patient and his family. Each of the stories in this book is really just a "lifebeat" in the overall picture of what it means to be a nurse. And that's what it's really all about.

i

Angel On His Shoulder

The kids were still little. They were all in the kitchen, that hot summer's day when the phone call came. Her husband was sick, the company nurse told her. He had been taken to the hospital. Anthony was only thirty-three years old.

She left the kids with a neighbor and took off for the emergency room. It was only about a mile away and she knew the fastest route there. After all, she had been working there in the I.C.U. of that hospital for almost ten years.

As she entered the E.R., she saw the ambulance just pulling up the ramp. She knew he was inside. As the squad wheeled past her, she looked at her husband. His color was gray and he was covered with sweat. His eyes were closed.

Elaine knew something was very wrong. All the nurse had told her on the phone was that he had collapsed, complaining of pain in his neck. She had thought at the time that the pain was in the front of his neck, and most likely from his chest.

But when she finally got to speak to him, he told her that he had felt some kind of a popping in his head and then the terrible pain in the back of his neck. Then he had vomited.

Elaine knew, just knew, that her husband had bled somewhere inside his head. It was the classic onset of a sub-arachnoid hemorrhage. She had been an I.C.U. nurse for too many years.

So the first thing they did was wheel him off for a CT scan. If he really had an intracerebral bleed, they told her, it would show up on the scan. And it really was lucky that their hospital had its own scanner. Back then, in 1979, many community hospitals had to send their patients out to big medical centers for CT's.

After what seemed like forever to Elaine, Anthony was brought back to the emergency room. Then they had to wait. Elaine thought she was going to faint, but she sat there just like all the families sat there, and she waited. And waited. Then the results came. No bleed. Nothing at all.

So after consulting with a neurologist, the decision was that this was some kind of a weird migraine and Anthony could go home. With a prescription for pain pills in her hand, Elaine left the emergency room and brought her car up to the ramp. Somehow Anthony, who could hardly walk, was helped into the car. And they drove home.

No matter what the doctors had told her, Elaine knew that something was not right. She still believed he had suffered a bleed. This was not a migraine. Anthony never had migraines. Somehow she managed to get him out of the car and up the front steps into the living room. Anthony collapsed onto the couch and fell into a deep sleep. Elaine remembers that his suit jacket was so drenched with perspiration that she could literally wring it out.

An hour later, Anthony was still sleeping. When she managed to wake him up, he was confused. He didn't know where he was. Elaine went to the phone and called the neurologist. They had known each other for years and he knew she wasn't the type to overreact. He told her to get Anthony back to the hospital and he would do a spinal tap the following morning.

The volunteer ambulance squad had to carry Anthony out on the stretcher. He barely responded to their questions. Anthony was admitted to Elaine's own unit. His nurses and his medical residents were her friends. Several hours later, Elaine went home, picked up her kids, and started making phone calls.

Elaine, who was on vacation at the time, arrived at her I.C.U. the first thing the next morning. She even beat the neurologist there. When the doctor arrived, he began to do the spinal tap. Elaine waited outside in the nurses' station. Just then her friend Lynne came through, saying they needed another spinal tap kit since the doctor had dropped something on the floor. It turned out later that the first tap had been so bloody, the doctor was sure he had gone directly into a blood vessel. He wanted to repeat it. When the second tap was the same, they had their diagnosis. Lynne took the fluid, which they described as looking like tomato juice, down to the lab the back way so that Elaine couldn't see the specimen.

And so the process began. The next day Anthony had a repeat CT scan, which showed the bleed. It was in the posterior fossa, an area which, in the imperfect beginnings of CT scanning, had been missed. Anthony had an angiogram four days later. It showed no aneurysm. A week later he had another angiogram, because there had to be a reason for a bleed this big, a reason that should show up. But once again they told her that the test was negative, and if he continued to improve, he could probably go home by the end of the week.

That afternoon, while the kids were in visiting their father, the neurologist called Elaine. He had just heard from the radiologist who had been going over and over those films, and they found it. There was an aneurysm in the back of the brain. If it wasn't repaired, he could very well re-bleed and die. Elaine remembers going into the little bathroom right off the nurses station and vomiting. The plans had changed from taking Anthony home to taking him to surgery. Her friend Lynne was once again with her.

Later on in the week Anthony had another spinal tap done to see if the amount of blood in the spinal fluid had decreased. He also had to have a third angiogram, since the neurosurgeon wanted to have different views to see which vessels fed into what. Lynne asked the surgeon if he thought Anthony should be moved to a bigger medical

2

enter for the surgery. The doctor told her that if he honestly believed that things would be better that way, he would be the first one to recommend it. Lynne had known this neurosurgeon for many years and she trusted him completely.

Three weeks after that first bleed, Anthony went off to the operating room. He had just gotten his preoperative demerol when he once again began to moan in pain, saying his head and neck were hurting. Elaine attributed it to a reaction to demerol.

She waited in the lobby all day. Anthony's family was with her. Thinking back now, she remembers that when Anthony first left for the O.R., she heard the code which invites any and all interested personnel to come watch a particular autopsy. Elaine had jumped, thinking it was Anthony, and then had laughed out loud when she realized how crazy a thought that was.

Eight hours later, Elaine was summoned to the information desk. The neurosurgeon told her it was all over and everything went well. Elaine remembers the exact words. She asked, "Is he going to be O.K.?" The doctor had replied, "I think so." The relief that Elaine felt was so overwhelming that it was more physical than emotional. She'll never forget the feeling.

Well, it turned out that the aneurysm had not had a "stem", so there was nothing to put a clamp on. Instead, the anethesioligist had purposely dropped Anthony's blood pressure, and then the neurosurgeon had coated the entire ballooned area of the artery with cyanoacrylic. That was a fancy name for Crazy Glue, which is exactly what Anthony, to this day, has in his brain.

As the assisting neurosurgeon later told Elaine, when Anthony is long gone in his grave, the Crazy Glue will still be there. So there would be no worry about it holding and keeping the area solid, preventing it from leaking ever again. Today, with the vast array of aneurysm clips available, there probably is one that would have fit. But not then.

More than sixteen years have gone by. Looking back now, Elaine, who is still a critical care nurse, can see so many things that could have gone wrong. But they didn't. Anthony had been sent home and he walked up those steps. He should have been kept absolutely quiet. But the stress did not cause a rebleed. A spinal tap is never done today when there is suspicion of an intra-cerebral bleed. Anthony had two. The brain could herniate down from the pressure. But it didn't.

Angiograms which are done when there is spasm present are very dangerous. Nobody mentioned spasm, maybe because they never found the area that had bled. Till later. Techniques were different then. And most of all, that pain which Anthony felt right after the shot of demerol turned out not to be from the medication. The surgeon told Elaine that Anthony had rebled immediately before the surgery, and probably right

3

then. The area had been full of fresh bright red blood and there was some spasm present. All direct and dangerous contraindications to surgery.

But Anthony sailed through it all. On his second post-operative day, he sat up in bed and did the New York Times crossword puzzle. He was discharged home on day six, and went back to work five weeks after that.

There is no reason or answer as to why things worked out as they did. Elaine just believes that it wasn't Anthony's time yet, and that there had to have been an angel on his shoulder watching over him. It took a very long time for Elaine to be able to talk about all of this. It was sort of a bad dream that she didn't want to remember. And many people told her to write a story about it. But she just couldn't.

Until now.

The Right Time and Place for a Miracle

It was just renal colic. Now anyone who has ever had an episode of renal colic does not use the word "just", since renal colic has been likened to giving birth. It hurts terribly.

But when you get down to the basics, renal colic occurs when the kidney or ureter goes into spasm while trying to pass a stone. And that, in itself, is not a fatal disease. As sick as the person gets, he or she will survive.

So on this particular evening, Jeffrey Boldin was in renal colic. He had been writhing around in pain at home for several hours before letting his wife take him to the hospital. And he only gave in after beginning to vomit non-stop. He thought he was dying. Well, the emergency department physician was reasonably sure of his diagnosis even before sending the patient over to x-ray for the I.V.P. The symptoms were classic. So they doped Jeffrey up with morphine and he finally fell asleep. The pictures were taken and now it was going to be a short wait for them to be officially read.

Jeffrey was returned to the holding area of the emergency room. His wife, Elaine, was with him as was their three year old son and infant daughter. Elaine had packed them all up and had taken them in the car with Jeffrey. She had nobody to leave the kids with, and so the trip to the emergency room had turned into a family affair. The little boy, Jimmy, was out in waiting area, which had plenty of toys to keep him busy. And Elaine was able to watch him from the doorway of the holding area. The baby, Chrissy, was fast asleep in her car bed, right there in the room with them.

About ten minutes later, Jimmy became bored and walked in to be with his mom and dad. He leaned over his sister, who seemed to be fast asleep. "Chrissy," he yelled at her, as he pulled back the blanket. "Wake up and play with me." Elaine took Jimmy by the hand and gently pulled him back from the car bed. "Don't bother Chrissy," she said, reaching to put the cover back over the baby. And then she froze. Something was wrong with Chrissy. Her color was chalky white and she wasn't breathing.

Elaine grabbed the baby and pulled her from the car bed. Chrissy's eyes were wide open, and her pupils were dilated. "Oh, my God," screamed Elaine. "Help me!" Before anyone could respond, Elaine ran toward the main nurses' station of the emergency department with the baby in her arms. Within seconds, Chrissy was grabbed by the nurses and they began to work on her. The baby was clinically dead. She had no heartbeat or respirations.

A pediatric code was called. Everyone who was supposed to respond did so. By this time Elaine had become hysterical, and Jeffrey had pulled out his I.V. and climbed off the stretcher. The little boy was screaming, knowing that something horrible was happening. And it was.

This was a small community hospital without a pediatric I.C.U., so plans were made immediately to transfer the baby out. But meanwhile, that baby was the priority of the emergency department staff. And as luck would have it, there was a doctor moonlighting there that evening who just happened to be a resident in anesthesiology. He intubated little Chrissy with no trouble and they began to breathe for her. And within ten minutes Chrissy's pulse and respiratory effort were back. Good and strong.

Well, the pediatric transport team arrived and they took her with them back to their pediatric center. Within a very short time, the baby was stable and alert. Someone took Jimmy to a neighbor's house and Mom and Dad drove the thirty miles to the other hospital to be with their baby. And as soon as they arrived there, Jeffrey went to the bathroom and passed his kidney stone.

So what took place? They called it an "interrupted S.I.D.S. death," a sudden infant death which was reversed only because of the circumstances. Chrissy did very well. She was discharged home within a few days on an apnea monitor, and is now a healthy toddler.

Many people say that all of what happened did so for a reason. Jeffrey developed his renal colic only so that his daughter would be in a hospital emergency room at the exact moment that she "died." And Jimmy picked that exact moment to come in an play with his sister. And it took place on the rare night that this particular anesthesiologist was present right there in the E.R. The fact that Jeffrey passed the stone as soon as the baby was O.K. meant that the stone had served its purpose, these same people say.

Some believe that all this is nonsense. It was just a stroke of good luck. Maybe so. But then again, who really knows for sure?

"The Right Time and Place for a Miracle", by Linda Strangio RN MA CCRN. From: *The Nursing Spectrum*, New York/New Jersey Metro Edition. Reprinted with permission.

Letting Go

She had lived with it for five years, and she now it was time. She didn't want to go on like that, even though she was only thirty years old.

A very rare type of cancer had been found deep in Lila's pelvis, and although various surgeries and treatments had slowed its growth, it never went away. And now it was growing. Growing very rapidly. The cancer did not travel through her bloodstream to distant organs as so many other types of cancer did, but it spread by direct extension throughout her pelvis and abdomen. It was everywhere. The tumors could be felt easily through Lila's skin. Cancers had attached themselves to the abdominal wall, so when she lay flat in bed, she looked as if she were covered with bumps.

The masses were solid and hard, and pushed on all of Lila's vital organs. Her bowels were partially obstructed and her liver, spleen, and pancreas were being moved up and away from where they belonged. Even Lila's kidneys were displaced. And there was fluid everywhere, which pushed up against her diaphragm and made it hard to breathe. The CT scans showed it all.

Lila lived at home with her mother and father. They took care of her. She existed with a nasogastric tube in place to keep her stomach from becoming too distended, since only minimal amounts of gastrointestinal contents were able to pass through her system. She had an implanted central venous line through which Lila received all her nourishment. The home care nurses had taught Lila and her parents to take care of it. She had adequate pain control with the patch she wore on her skin.

But Lila's parents refused to accept the fact that Lila wasn't going to get better. They often talked about the time when she'd be able to eat again. That's when she'd get her strength back and feel better, they seemed to believe. Lila only nodded.

Lila made frequent visits to the hospital. She needed more and more paracenteses to drain the increasing amounts of abdominal fluid which accumulated inside her. And because of the multiple areas of solid tumor masses, she needed to be drained by CT scan or ultrasound guidance. Otherwise, the doctors had no way of knowing if they were placing their needles into pockets of fluid or into areas of cancer growth.

Lila, through all of this, stayed sweet and outwardly cheerful. In between the bouts of vomiting right around her tube, she'd smile and say things like, "Oh, boy, look at me. I must look terrible." Lila had big bright eyes and when she smiled, they lit up.

7

As sick as she was, she was still very beautiful. She always took care of herself and kept her hair and makeup perfect.

It was only when Lila was alone, away from her parents, that she opened up. She told the nurses that she considered it nothing short of a miracle that she was still alive, since five years ago the doctors told her she only had one to two years to live. And, she added, she couldn't take away her parents' hope. That was all they had left. When it got really hard, she thought of her mother and father and what it must be like for them. And then she pushed any thoughts of giving up out of her mind. She had to. She couldn't do that to her parents.

The months passed and Lila got worse. Even with the tube draining her stomach, she continued to have bouts of vomiting. She vomited bile, which seemed to come straight from her small intestine. The obstructions were getting worse. But she stayed home with her parents. One of them was always with her; Lila was never left alone. There was no talk of Hospice, since they did not even seem to consider the possibility that she was dying.

One evening while Lila was sleeping, her breathing seemed to get slower and slower. And then it stopped. Lila's father gave her mouth to mouth resuscitation while her mother called 911. The paramedics came to the house and intubated her. Lila was taken to the hospital, where she was put on a respirator and brought up to the I.C.U. There was no question that everything humanly possible was to be done. That's what the parents wanted.

After two days, Lila's breathing was strong enough so that she could be taken off the respirator. When her parents left the room, Lila told the nurses that "we had a dress rehearsal for the real thing. I think it's time to tell my parents that the main event is not too far away."

Lila went home with her parents. Nobody really knows what happened then, except that Lila's doctors were informed that there was to be no more treatment and no more trips to the hospital. Lila sent a message that she wanted to thank everyone for all their support and understanding and for backing her up with whatever choices she had made over the past months. And she wanted to say goodbye to everyone.

Lila died a week later. Not one person ever said that things should have happened differently, or that her parents were right or wrong, or that Lila could have said this or done that to them. And that's kind of amazing, since nurses usually have opinions on these kinds of things. But in this case, it was very simple. Lila had to be in charge. She let things stay the way they were until she felt she was completely ready. She did it her way.

The Mouthpiece

It had been one of those days. It had poured all night and into the morning, which had put everyone in bad moods. Nothing had gone right and everything had gone wrong. The phone was never silent, the call bells never stopped, and the visitors were unhappy about almost everything. Doctors complained, supplies were missing, medications arrived late, and only part of the linen supply came up. It had been an ugly shift and Barbara couldn't wait to go home.

Her jaw was hurting again. Barbara had been diagnosed with temporomandibular joint syndrome, which became aggravated every time she was stressed. Her doctor told her she must be subconsciously biting down or tensing her jaw muscles, which increased the spasm and pain in that area. She needed to relax. The specially made mouthpiece really did help, but for obvious reasons she couldn't wear it at work. She usually stuck it in her mouth at night, when she was home relaxing.

By the time Barbara left the hospital, the sun had come up and the hot and humid summer air was being replaced by a cool and dry breeze. Maybe she could save some of this day after all, Barbara thought. After all, it was still the afternoon.

Barbara stopped off at the supermarket and did her food shopping. She unpacked and put away her groceries and made herself a hamburger. By the time she had cleaned up the kitchen, it was just six o'clock. And the evening had become really beautiful.

After taking a shower and washing her hair, Barbara decided that she would go sit outside in her backyard and read the paper. Nobody could see her, she knew, since the trees and bushes really hid the yard from the street and from the view of her neighbors. So clad only in her nightgown, Barbara trotted outside with the newspaper and a radio under one arm and a cold beer under the other. The fact that the nightgown was sort of "see-through" never bothered her. She knew she was all alone, sitting there in a lawn chair with her soaking wet hair dripping all over and her very ugly retainer sticking out of her mouth. Nobody would ever know.

Yeah, right.

About ten minutes later, Barbara heard a man's voice. "Yoo, hoo," it called out. "I thought you were out there!" Barbara froze in her seat. Then the man appeared around the back of the house. It was the Rabbi who lived down the block. "I was

taking a little walk," he said, "and I thought we could talk for a while. It's such a nic
night."

Barbara, realizing that this man could see right through her nightgown, didn
know what to do. She had nothing to cover herself with and knew that if she stood up
the sunlight would stream right through the sheer nightgown, giving the Rabbi a perfec
show. So, as she always did when she got nervous, Barbara tensed up all her muscles
including those in her jaw.

Just at that minute, Barbara was conscious of something glinting and flashing.
The only problem was that this flickering was coming from the Rabbi's pants. To be
exact, it was originating in his crotch. Barbara couldn't help it. Her eyes kept darting
down there. It was as if the Rabbi was sending her a signal from his crotch. Was she
losing her mind? Suddenly she realized that the man had a safety pin down at the
bottom of his zipper. A tiny gold one, which was picking up the rays of sunshine as the
leaves on the trees moved in the soft evening breeze. Barbara could not control her
eyes. It was as if the zipper was sending her a message in Morse Code. She kept
glancing down at his crotch and then pulling her eyes away. She couldn't stop herself.

As Barbara tried to smile politely at the Rabbi, she began to salivate. Profusely.
The saliva dripped out of her mouth and down her chin. As she frantically grabbed for
the napkin she had rested her beer bottle on, she dumped the beer onto the Rabbi's foot.
Torn between mopping at his beer soaked shoe or trying to slow the torrent of saliva
running from her mouth down the front of her peek-a-boo nightgown, she first dabbed
wildly at her chin. Then, without thinking, Barbara leaned over and, with the saliva
coated napkin, began to swipe at the Rabbi's foot.

The Rabbi, by this time, appeared stunned. He stood up, just at the exact
moment that Barbara did the same. Trying to cover herself with both hands, she
knocked the dripping wet retainer from her mouth. It bounced off his glistening crotch,
landing on his beer drenched shoe.

"Oh, excuse me, Rabbi," mumbled Barbara, her face bright red. Then she
became almost aphasic, the only sound coming from her salivating mouth being, "Heh,
heh, heh." The Rabbi suddenly realized that this dripping wet person who had been
staring at his crotch for the last few minutes was stark naked under her nightgown. He
decided it was time to leave. And fast. His face, by this time, was almost as red as
Barbara's. "Good night," he whispered hoarsely, as he bolted from the back yard.

Barbara, now fully aware that her only recourse was to sell her house, quit her
job, and move away from this neighborhood, grabbed the dirty retainer. She rolled it up
in the newspaper, picked up the radio and the beer bottle, and fled to the safety of the
house. She was totally mortified.

Well, Barbara went to bed, and after tossing and turning for quite a while, she finally was able to fall asleep. At about two in the morning, while having some kind of a crazy dream, Barbara was awakened by loud screeching noises. Looking out of the window, she saw a cat which appeared to be fighting with a bunch of birds. For whatever reason, Barbara suddenly remembered that she had no idea what she had done with her retainer after she had rolled it up in the newspaper. She had never put it away or washed it off. Well, Barbara thought, the mouthpiece would have to wait. First she had to see what was happening in her yard.

So out the door flew Barbara, clutching a flashlight. She was disgusted by what she saw. A stray cat was in the process of tearing a bird apart, while what seemed like a thousand other birds screeched in protest. Without a second's hesitation, Barbara grabbed the garden hose and took aim at the cat. The force of the stream of water hit the obviously dead bird, as well as startling the cat and making it let go. The cat ran away, leaving the mass of hovering birds behind. Almost immediately, the flock took off and headed for the trees above. Barbara, watching them go, saw her mouthpiece clutched in the claws of one of the larger birds. It had obviously fallen from the rolled up paper and the bird had found it and was taking it away with him.

Barbara, having no idea what she was doing, sprayed that garden hose at the mass of birds, screaming out loud, "Bring back my retainer, you horrible birds!" Her mouthpiece disappeared into the night, leaving Barbara standing there soaking wet in her see-through nightgown. By this time, she could hear the neighbors at their windows and doors. Barbara ran into her house, knowing this was the end. She would definitely have to move away, and fast.

Well, Barbara was never able to get back to sleep that night, and before she knew it, it was time to get up and go to back to the hospital. She called her doctor to tell him she needed another mouthpiece. Being the honest person she always was, she told the doctor the truth. A bird had flown away with her original one. "Barbara," the doctor quietly asked, "What kind of drugs are you taking?"

So the order was placed and the replacement retainer was made. It arrived, naturally, on the same day that Barbara found her first one on the ground in the backyard, where the bird had dropped it out of the tree after realizing it wasn't something to eat. The Rabbi began crossing the street whenever he had to go near Barbara's house. Although she never put her house up for sale, she had less and less contact with the neighbors, who obviously decided that some kind of lunatic nurse was living amongst them. Barbara does not go outside in her nightgown any more, and she alternates regularly between her two retainers. Indoors.

The Panty Hose

Look at that foley bag, thought Jane. Urine was dripping right from where the
plastic drain hooks into the holder, and there was, in fact, quite a puddle on the floor.
Obviously, the last person to empty that bag never closed the metal clamp tightly.
Sloppy.

Jane was on the phone with the hospital operator at the time, waiting while she
checked on a phone number. The small I.C.U. was quiet, with only two of the four
beds filled. And while Jane waited, an alarm on one of the two respirators started to
sound. From where Jane stood she could see what it was; the tubing had popped off the
trach. She could hook that back up before the operator even came back on the phone,
Jane was sure. So she laid the phone on the counter and zipped over to the patient's
bedside.

Jane connected the ventilator tubing to the blue adaptor and waited until the
alarm stopped. Then she ran back around the bed towards the phone. Coming around
the foot of the bed, Jane turned the corner sharply. She felt herself beginning to slide,
and before she could grab onto anything, she hit the floor. As she went down, her leg
turned sideways. Jane heard the crack almost before she felt the pain.

And then Jane, who was alone in the unit, screamed out loud. She couldn't help
it. She felt the bones moving in her leg as she tried to straighten it out. She heard them
crunch and she knew her leg was broken. Suddenly, Jane heard the overhead page
calling the code team. Instinctively, she tried to get up, thinking she had to respond to
wherever the cardiac arrest was. And then she realized that the operator was calling the
team to her I.C.U. Jane looked toward the desk and saw the telephone receiver lying
there, on top of a bunch of papers. Jane knew what had happened. The operator, who
had obviously come back on the phone, had heard Jane screaming, and was sending the
cavalry to save her.

A few seconds later, the nurses' aide ran into the unit. Her eyes skimmed the
room and came to rest on Jane, who was lying at the side of the bed, her leg bent at a
crazy angle. "Honey," the aide asked seriously. "What the hell are you doing on the
floor?" Jane closed her eyes and groaned. "I think I broke my leg," she answered in a
tiny little voice.

By the time the mob of people descended on the I.C.U., Jane was totally and
profoundly mortified. The aide had brought a big plastic bag filled with crushed ice

and plopped it on top of Jane's twisted and rapidly swelling leg. But what bothered Jan
the most was the fact that she was soaked in urine, the urine which had leaked from the
partially open foley bag. And it was the smelly infected urine of an old lady with a
urinary tract infection. Every nurse knows what that smells like. And Jane knew better
than just any nurse; after all, she was lying in it.

Well, two orderlies appeared and they rolled Jane onto a blanket and lifted her up
into one of her own empty beds. An orthopedist appeared from nowhere and examined
her right then and there. It was obvious to him, even without an x-ray, that it was a bad
break. "You're going to be out of work for some time," he announced with a smile.
"You really did a nice job on this."

Jane did not smile back, because by now she was becoming angry. She was
starting to realize just what had really happened to her just because a nurse had been
careless with the clamp on a foley bag. She had a lot of things she had to do. She didn't
have the time to be laid up with a broken leg. This wasn't fair. If she had fallen on the
ice or had been in a car accident, well, maybe. But to have taken a flying leap onto pee
from a leaky foley bag because some nurse was too lazy to fasten the clip? Oh, boy.
Now Jane was getting madder.

By this time, Jane's friend Nancy was at the bedside, trying to cut off Jane's
soaking wet panty hose with her trusty bandage scissors. Obviously, it was the thing to
do since it didn't look as if Jane would appreciate the pulling and tugging it takes to
remove panty hose. But Nancy didn't count on Jane being a raving maniac. "You're not
cutting off these panty hose!" Jane screamed, waving her arms like a helicopter
propeller. "These panty hose cost me $5.95 in Macy's and you're not going to ruin
them. It's enough that they will probably smell like old lady pee forever. They can take
the damn x-rays right through them."

The orthopedist walked up to Jane. "You are obviously in pain," he said, trying
to be kind. "I'll see that you get a shot of demerol." Jane glared at him, her face
becoming redder and redder. "I don't want any damn demerol," she said quietly. "Oh,
O.K.," said the doctor. "How about some codeine?" Jane started to scream. "Don't
patronize me! I don't want any codeine!" She pulled her pillow off the bed and threw it
on the floor, and then did the same with the box of tissues on the bedside table. By this
time, the doctor was getting a little impatient. "Then how about some valium?" he
suggested sarcastically. Jane went nuts. "I don't want drugs! I want a bath! I'm
covered with smelly disgusting old lady pee! Get out of here!" The doctor left the unit.

After her x-rays, Jane was transferred up to a regular floor and they put her in a
private room. She told everyone to get out and leave her alone, even though she was
still in her damp urine soaked uniform and those soggy $5.95 panty hose. As soon as
she was alone, Jane slid out of the bed. She grabbed the clean gown which had been

13

left on the chair, and hopped across the room to the bathroom. And with her freshly broken and uncasted unsplinted leg complete with its unstable slipping and sliding bones, Jane took a shower and washed her hair. She then hopped back to the bed and pulled off the sheets which had been in contact with the old lady pee soaked clothes, threw them on the floor, and made her bed with the linen that she found stashed in the closet. Then she got into bed. A little part of her was sorry she hadn't fallen again and hurt herself worse because then they would have had to write out an incident report about how they could have let a patient with broken bones take a shower and make her bed all by herself. Jane hated everyone.

Well, it took Jane a couple of days to calm down. Her friend Nancy actually brought her a tennis ball which she continuously threw against the wall and caught. It was either that, said Nancy, or she would be bouncing herself off the wall. The first thing Jane did when she went home was to wash those stinky clothes in detergent and clorox, and in no time they smelled fresh and clean again.

And as they say, the best medicine can be a dose of tincture of time. She never said a word to the nurse who had left the foley bag clamp open. Jane's leg healed and so did her anger, and the very first day she came back to work she wore those $5.95 panty hose, washed and clean and still in one piece.

Carrot Tops

It was her second delivery, and her first had been a piece of cake. The whole labor had lasted under two hours and she had given birth to a beautiful baby girl. The delivery staff remembered this patient, because her baby had the same orange colored hair as she did.

So this time, they were waiting to see another carrot top kid come out. Wanda knew she was having a boy, and a big one at that. The ultrasound had told them.

Wanda received her epidural, and she felt very comfortable. Delivery was imminent. Suddenly, Wanda developed chest pain. She broke out into a cold sweat and said she couldn't breathe. And her color was horrible.

STAT calls went out to everyone to help the O.B. team. The different specialists responded immediately, all with a sick feeling inside. This shouldn't be happening. The cardiogram showed lots of premature beats and strongly indicated that Wanda, right in the middle of having a baby, was also having a heart attack.

This baby had to come out. The infarcting heart could not handle the stress of labor, but it was too late to do a C-section. The head was crowning and Wanda's pain was getting worse and her breathing was more and more labored. The delivery team held its breath as the baby emerged. The little boy, it's orange hair matted down flat, gave a big yell. He was fine.

Almost as soon as the placenta was expelled, Wanda started to feel better. The pain began to quickly ease up, even before the nitroglycerin drip was hung. And almost miraculously, Wanda's E.K.G. changes resolved. The cardiac pattern was now almost normal. She was going to be fine. Everyone gave a sigh of relief. A patient who had just delivered a baby could not receive T.P.A., the wonder "clotbuster" drug. She could bleed to death. And now she didn't need it.

An emergency echocardiogram was done and it showed that Wanda did have a reduced ejection fraction. And the cardiac enzymes in her blood were elevated. Her heart, indeed, had been affected. But what had happened? Why, in the middle of a delivery, would a healthy young woman have a heart attack?

They had few ideas and no answers. A cardiac catheterization was done a few days later, and they found that Wanda's coronary arteries were perfectly normal. They were wide open. Then how and why could she infarct? A literature search was done as the computer helped the doctors search for an answer. And they finally found it.

The epinephrine in the epidural analgesia must have caused spasm in Wanda's coronary arteries. The coronaries, big as they are, are blood vessels just like those in the legs. And as a person might develop a cramp in his legs caused by a temporary decrease in blood supply to the leg muscle, Wanda developed a cramp in the arteries bringing blood to the muscle in the heart. For whatever reason, the epinephrine caused the vessels to contract too much. And that part of the heart, deprived of blood for even a short time, died.

Well, Wanda did very well. She was discharged home in less than a week. Her heart, with its normal coronary arteries, picked up just where it left off, apparently doing very well without that small area which had been involved. And Wanda went on with her happy and healthy life, taking care of her herself, her husband, and her two carrot topped babies. And they all lived happily ever after.

Mrs. Merkel's Family

Mrs. Merkel had been in the intensive care unit for more than a week. She'd had some type of intestinal surgery and then developed several abscesses in her abdominal cavity. Mrs. Merkel was a big fat lady, or as it said in the chart, she was "morbidly obese." Her size made her prone to many complications, and she'd been back to the operating room twice since the initial surgery. She was still running high fevers and had a very high white blood count. Rita, the I.C.U. head nurse, guessed that Mrs. Merkel had a long road ahead of her still, possibly with more surgery ahead. Since she worked the day shift and left by mid afternoon, Rita had never met Mrs. Merkel's family. They only visited at night, but their time in the hospital certainly left an impression. It seems that Mrs. Merkel's family hated everything about this hospital and everyone who worked in it. All they did was complain. In fact, that very morning Rita had gotten a note from one of the evening nurses saying that the family wanted to speak to Rita about the care, or lack of it, which was being given to Mrs. Merkel. Oh, great, Rita thought. Terrific. Something to look forward to.

Shortly after one that afternoon, Rita returned from the cafeteria where she had just eaten her favorite meal: a cholesterol burger (as she called it) and french fries. Forget all this healthy heart stuff and those people who delicately dab at their tuna fish piled on lettuce leaves. Some day, Rita thought, maybe she'd look just like Mrs. Merkel. But as for now, she was just fine.

There were two people standing at the nurses' station, apparently waiting for Rita to return from lunch. One of them looked at her as she approached, then pointedly looked at his watch. He was obviously annoyed that she had taken a lunch break. Rita immediately found herself becoming defensive. This is going to be a problem, she said to herself, knowing instinctively that these people were here to register a complaint. She was wrong. They were here to register a multitude of complaints, and they were, of course, Mrs. Merkel's family.

It seemed they were so upset about the "terrible nursing care" that they just had to take time off from work to come in person and see the manager of this "so called intensive care unit." Rita counted to ten and told herself to stay calm. She listened to them ramble on and on about the "cold uncaring nurses who kept Mrs. Merkel in pain, and were so rough when they turned her, and made her wash her own face, and kept waking her up when she finally fell asleep, and didn't know what they were doing when

17

they tried to restart her I.V.'s, and pushed tubes up and down her nose." And so on, a
so on, and so on.

Rita, knowing that part of her head nurse role was to be a politician, simp
listened. She wanted to yell at them that the patient was a whiny annoying woman wł
never cooperated in her care and expected to lie there as if she were totally paralyze
and have everybody do everything for her. She wanted to tell them that one of tł
reasons she was sick and had so many complications was that she was too fat and nev
took care of herself while she was healthy, letting her diabetes and blood pressu
become totally out of control. She wanted to let them know how this lady scream
when someone simply moved her arm to take her blood pressure or straighten the shee
She wished she could describe the scene when it was time to simply help her turn ov
in bed.

But of course she couldn't do that. Instead, Rita bit her tongue and did what sł
was supposed to do. She attempted to explain why it was important for Mrs. Merkel
move about and use her own energy, rather than have everything done for her. She trie
to differentiate between pain and discomfort and the reason why Mrs. Merkel did hav
some discomfort at times. And then she had to do the hardest part; she had to apologiz
to the family on behalf of the unit for any perception of rudeness or uncaring that Mr
Merkel or the family may have experienced. Rita told them that before she left for tł
day, she would be sure to have a long talk with Mrs. Merkel, assuring her that he
complaints were being addressed. Seemingly satisfied, the family left to go home.
small part of Rita wanted to yell out after them that they were as obnoxious as Mr
Merkel was, and she could see why the evening shift couldn't stand them. Actually,
wasn't such a small part of her after all.

It was just after three in the afternoon. Rita was in the chart room going ov
change of shift report with the oncoming staff. Suddenly, an alarm sounded on one
the cardiac monitor banks. The nurses glanced over, unconcerned, since most alarm
were caused by interference or patients moving. The light over room 205 was flashin
however, and the screen showed a picture of the lethal arrhythmia, ventricul:
fibrillation. Room 205, naturally, was Mrs. Merkel's room.

The nurses dropped what they were doing and ran from the chart room, all full
aware that Mrs. Merkel would die within minutes unless this deadly rhythm wa
terminated. Tom, the evening charge nurse, grabbed the crash cart and pulled it wił
him. He was the only male nurse this I.C.U. had, and was often mistaken for a docto
Tom, however, was always quick to say, "I only wish I made the bucks the docto
make, but I'm proud to say that I am a nurse." He was a good guy.

Anyway, the first thing the nurses did was check the patient, since there had bee
more than a few times that codes were called and people started going a little crazy fc

18

hat simply was a problem with the monitoring system, sometimes known as "the loose ad syndrome." But this time it was for real. They pressed the button which ztomatically signaled a cardiac arrest code.

Tom and Rita, along with one other nurse, lifted Mrs. Merkel enough to slide to ardiac board under her back, and that in itself was no easy job. But they got it under aere just enough to keep her from bouncing against the soft mattress during the cardiac ampressions. Rita pulled down Mrs. Merkel's gown and pushed aside her monitoring ads. Tom opened a package of defibrillator pads and placed one of them over the anter of her chest and the other just below and to the left of her heart.

By the time the cardiac arrest team arrived, Mrs. Merkel had already been afibrillated several times. No good. She was still in v-fib. The code went on, C.P.R., rugs, shock. And again. And again. By this time, Mrs. Merkel's heart had stopped brillating. As a matter of fact, it had stopped doing anything. There was a straight line n the cardiac monitor and Mrs. Merkel was obviously dead. As a last resort, the urgical resident did a pericardial tap, sticking a needle directly into the sac around the eart. The blood that he drew back into the syringe formed a clot, which showed that a ericardial tamponade was not the cause of her trouble. The monitor continued to show straight line, and five minutes later, the code was called. Mrs. Merkel was ronounced dead at three forty-five in the afternoon.

"Oh, boy," sighed Rita. "This lady's family is going to positively freak out when ney are told she is dead. There is no doubt that they are going to blame us for this ome way, and say that we killed her." The staff knew, of course, that Rita was right.

One of the residents put out a call to Mrs. Merkel's private surgeon first. Dr. 3allman was the absolute favorite of all the nurses. Not only was he a marvelous urgeon, but he was a kind and compassionate person. He cared about the patients, heir families, and the nursing staff. Everyone loved to take care of Dr. Ballman's atients; he treated the nurses with consideration and respect and consulted with them ike true colleagues. It was too bad that as the attending surgeon in charge of the case, it vas up to him to call that crazy family and let them know that Mrs. Merkel had died. Ie was going to have to take the heat and listen to all the yelling and screaming.

Dr. Ballman called back a few minutes later. "Watch out, guys," he sighed. The daughter went nuts on me and she is already on her way to the hospital, dragging aer husband and brother with her. She is demanding an autopsy because she says she vants to know exactly what we did to cause her mother's death. She was screaming hat we'd better not touch her mother until she gets here, and I"m sure she probably hinks we will try to cover something up. Get ready for this nut case; she's a raging naniac." Rita hung up the phone and ran into the room to clean up the mess. All the laughter had to do was see tubes and blood and stuff all over and she'd be looking for a

butcher knife or something as the murder weapon. Tom pushed the crash cart out in th
hall and away from where the family would see it when they first came into the unit
Under ordinary circumstances, it probably was a good thing to show a family just ho
hard people had tried to save the patient, but not in this case. Tom was sure that th
looney daughter would probably see the equipment as instruments used to hurt Mr
Merkel, and not to help her.

Tom looked at the chart to see if he could find the daughter's address so as to ti
to see just how long it would take for them to get to the hospital. He guessed not mor
than twenty minutes, and maybe less. He had a vision of the daughter being stopped fc
speeding and her telling the cop that she was racing to the hospital because her mothe
had just been murdered. She'd probably wind up getting a police escort.

Twenty minutes later, almost to the dot, the big double doors to the unit flev
open and Mrs. Merkel's daughter ran in, sobbing out loud and screaming for her mothe
Instinctively, all three of the nurses flew into the chart room, as if to get away from wha
was yet to come. They could hear the crying and moaning becoming louder, an
through the glass windows of the room they could see the daughter pacing around an
around. Taking a deep breath, Rita left the chart room and walked slowly into roor
205. The daughter was leaning over the body of her mother and was kissing her face.

Rita spoke first, telling the daughter that Mrs. Merkel had developed a sudde
deadly heart rhythm. She stressed that this had been found at the second it developec
and that everything possible had been done to reverse the rhythm and try to save th
patient. She spoke quietly and compassionately with the intent to convey the idea tha
there was nothing at all that could have been done to prevent this catastrophic event.
And all of this was true. Mrs. Merkel's daughter said nothing to Rita for a while. Sh
continued to hold on to the body and stroke her mother's face and hair. The other twc
family members simply stood in the corner of the room, quietly looking at what th
daughter was doing.

Suddenly the daughter became aware that Rita was in the room, and that she hac
been talking to her. Obviously the daughter had not heard one word of what had beer
said, because she looked quickly up at Rita as if she were seeing her for the first time.
She said, "You! All of you nurses are responsible for what happened to my mother.
There was no reason for her to die. She died because of your negligence. You treatec
her horribly and caused her pain and agony for the last week and a half. You were al
probably out on one of your many coffee breaks while all of this was happening. Well
I'm calling my lawyer the first thing in the morning and you can bet that all your asses
will be sued. You will all pay dearly for what you did."

Rita turned around and stormed out of the room. She just couldn't deal with this
bitch any more, and she was well aware that anything she might say would only make

20

hings worse. Thank God her shift was over, she thought, because she just couldn't unction any more. She needed to leave the hospital. Right now.

And she did.

Big Tommy

It all happened early that Saturday morning before she came in to work, but as soon as she walked through the doors she knew there was going to be a problem. Connie was filling in as nursing supervisor that weekend and so it became her headache.

Big Tommy, as he was called around the neighborhood, was dead. Everyone knew Big Tommy, since he weighed in at about five hundred pounds or so. Tommy had a family, but lived mostly on the streets. He didn't get along with a lot of people, and had many problems. Tommy's health had been poor for the past year or so. He was a regular in the emergency room, and never listened to medical advice. He was a non-compliant diabetic and had multiple leg ulcers which he wouldn't, or couldn't, take care of.

Well, this time Tommy had been admitted with sepsis and had coded just a few hours after he was brought up to the floor. Because of his size, Big Tommy had been put in a private room, and this really had turned out to be a blessing. According to the night staff, the entire code had turned out to be a circus.

Due to the amount of fat on his arms, nobody had been able to get an I.V. line into him, and when his heart stopped, getting I.V. access became the priority. Well, Big Tommy was stuck over and over again by almost everyone in the room. No luck. So of course the residents tried to get a central line in. That was fine, except for one minor problem. His chest and his neck were also lined with layers of fat.

The long needles just could not get down to the subclavian veins or into his jugulars. They tried to give intracardiac adrenalin, but the same situation existed there. There was too much fat for them to reach his heart. So Big Tommy died.

This particular Saturday was the second week of August, right smack in the dog days of one of the hottest summers on record. And Tommy's nursing unit was in the oldest building in the hospital, where the air conditioning system worked only occasionally. Naturally, this was one of the times when the system was down. And as luck would have it, the curtains on the windows of Big Tommy's room would not close. So the hot summer sun beat in through those big glass windows, raising the temperature in the room and making it very uncomfortable for everyone.

When Connie finally got up to the nursing unit that morning, Big Tommy had been dead for over three hours. His body was still in the bed, because it was obvious that it would never fit in a morgue refrigerator. They realized that when they had first

22

attempted to wrap it for the morgue and found the shroud pack too small. So Conni
went into that overheated room to see Big Tommy's body and it was then that she firs
began to smell something funny.

Now even though bodies are really supposed to be sent down to the morgu
within an hour of being pronounced dead, that doesn't always happen. And it doesn
really make that much of a difference. But in this case it certainly did. At first the
weren't sure what the smell was, but then they realized what had happened.

Between the I.V. tries and the attempts to reach his major blood vessels an
heart, Big Tommy probably had been stuck close to fifty times. And C.P.R. was i
progress at the time, pumping his blood throughout the body. So all those needle hole
had leaked blood which had dripped out and run over his arms and chest and ha
pooled under him. Big Tommy's mammoth body was covering a huge pool of blooc
which in the heat of the room and under the weight of his body, was beginning t
putrefy.

Connie knew that this body couldn't remain where it was much longer. In thi
particular hospital, the nursing floors simply contacted the Admitting Department whe
someone died, and the funeral directors dealt directly with Admitting when they arrive
to pick the bodies up from the morgue. The floors and the nursing supervisors had n
contact at all with the funeral homes. So the first thing Connie did was to try to find ou
which funeral home had been called by Tommy's family. When she found tha
Admitting hadn't been contacted as of yet, Connie decided that she needed to ge
involved.

She called the next of kin listed on Big Tommy's chart and matter of factly aske
them who they had called. Tommy's family assumed this was the way things normall
were done. Then Connie called the funeral director herself. Obviously, he had no ide
as to the size of the body, since he sort of lost it when Connie told him. She als
informed him that he'd better come soon, since Big Tommy was now beginning t
decompose in an overheated room on top of a big ocean of rotting blood.

Well, two hours later, three men arrived on the nursing unit. They had tap
measures and pads and pencils and they could be heard cursing and stamping inside Bi
Tommy's foul-smelling room. It was obvious that they were trying to figure out jus
how they were going to attempt to get that big body out of there.

Then suddenly, the men disappeared. They never said a word to anyone, bu
they just walked out. The floor nurses called Connie to say there was nobody left in Bi
Tommy's room but Big Tommy. And he was smelling pretty badly by now.

It was a good seven hours after Big Tommy had died when the undertaker
returned to the floor. They had the morgue orderly with them, who they obviousl
knew very well from all their routine visits to the hospital. And they were wheeling th

egulation morgue stretcher with them. Everyone except the orderly appeared annoyed
nd somewhat angry. The orderly obviously thought the situation was very funny.

Connie felt as if it were her duty to supervise this whole operation, which was a
oke since she had no idea what they were going to do or how they were going to do it.
ut she stayed there and watched, making sure that she was out of the way. The only
me she was addressed directly was when one of the funeral directors asked her if she
ould call a few more orderlies to help them.

Well, all the men put on patient gowns and rubber gloves and somehow they
managed to drag Big Tommy's body out of that smelly soaking wet bed and onto the
morgue stretcher. The heat of the room and the effort of the move left all the men
weaty and red faced. The body was balanced in the center of the stretcher with the tag
ed to the big toe. A clean sheet covered the huge mound on top of the stretcher, but
eftover blood trickled down one of the sides and over the wheels as it rolled.

The group of men steered the stretcher, which by this time was listing to the left,
ut of the unit and down the hall. There was absolute silence except for one half-
entence uttered by one of the funeral directors - - "If I had known it was this guy - - ".
And there was Connie, trailing behind the pack like some type of caboose. She spoke
only once, saying "Where are we going?" After a long look, she was answered. "To
he loading dock."

The parade attracted quite a few people, but Connie really doubted they knew
here was a dead body under the sheet, unless of course they noticed the trail of blood.
t looked like maybe a big mound of laundry or something. Connie's one fear was that
he stretcher was going to collapse and Big Tommy would splatter to the floor. She
emembered years back when she and a morgue orderly were moving a body from a
ed to the morgue stretcher and they had dropped it. She would never forget that
orrible noise when it hit the ground. And this body was at least three times as heavy.

When they finally made it to the loading dock, Connie realized that there was no
earse there. She had just assumed there would be. Instead there was a station wagon
arked with the tailgate open. There were no seats or anything in the back, and it was
bvious that it was waiting for Big Tommy. So the men heaved and pushed and
weated and managed to get that big body into the car.

That was it. The morgue orderly turned, and with a laugh he walked back into
he hospital with his blood stained stretcher. Two of the men got into another car and
ne got into the front of the station wagon. And they were gone. Connie wondered just
ow they were going to get Big Tommy's body out of the car and into the funeral home,
nd if they were going to have to bury him in a special coffin. It also crossed her mind
hat this funeral was probably going to be pretty expensive. But that stuff really wasn't
er business.

When Connie returned to the nursing floor, she found the room had bee stripped. The nurses told her they had taken the stinky sheets and thrown them into bi plastic bags to be thrown out with the trash. That was just fine, Connie told them Good thinking. The bed itself had been scrubbed, but the room still smelled horrible The housekeeper, wearing a mask, was scrubbing the floor. It was so warm in the that it was likely the odor would last a while. And of course, the bed was alread booked for the next patient.

Connie sighed as she left the unit. The new patient should only know what wa in his bed just a few hours earlier. Gross.

The Bun

It was a real miracle, they all said, that the lady had been found alive. She had been on the floor for a very long time. She was unconscious, and was covered with dog feces.

It seems that Mrs. Petrocelli had a little dog, who had been her constant companion. The dog must have been beside himself when his mistress had that stroke and there was nobody else around. Just the poor little lady and that poor little dog. By the dates on the mail which had been pushed through the slot in the door, the police figured that she had lain there for almost six days. When they had finally arrived at the house and had looked in through the window, they saw the dog lying on top of the lady, not understanding why she wouldn't wake up. The theory was that the dog had survived by drinking water from the toilet. Maybe it was due to panic or whatever, but the dog had defecated all over the lady. For six days straight.

Well, the dog was taken in by the neighbors and Mrs. Petrocelli was brought to the emergency department. Besides the feces, she was covered with sores, both from the pressure of lying in the one position as well as from the festering dog droppings which coated her body. The smell from this unfortunate lady filtered throughout the whole emergency room.

By the time Mrs. Petrocelli was brought up to the unit, she had been bathed and powdered. The E.R. nurses did a great job. The one remaining problem was her hair. You see, Mrs. Petrocelli was known around town as an eccentric old lady, and one of her eccentricities was her hair. She hadn't had a haircut for probably thirty years, and she wore her long mane pinned up on her head in a bun with a hundred or so hairpins holding it in place. The bun itself probably weighed a few pounds, and as you've probably guessed, it was matted solid with dog doo. The paper operating room cap covering that big loaded bun did very little to mask the stench.

This was a unique nursing problem, to say the least. Every nurse knows you just don't cut people's hair off. Not even a trim, at least not without written consent. But as Toni put it, "I'm doing what I have to do and that's the end of it." So "Project Bun" began. Mrs. Petrocelli, although comatose, was breathing very well on her own. She had an I.V. in place and a foley catheter, but that was all.

Toni decided that the first thing that this lady needed was a bath. A real tub bath. That was the priority. Now, giving real tub baths to I.C.U. patients was not exactly a

26

routine procedure. In fact, nobody even could remember when and if that old tub room had ever been used for anything but storage. So the first thing Toni did, even though she certainly had other patients to worry about, was to scrub the bathtub out. No big deal, said Toni. Just like home.

The tub was filled half way with warm water and a some of the bubble bath that one of the nurses had bought to freshen up the bath basins of her patients. Toni got dressed in O.R. scrubs, a hat, booties, and gloves. She looked as if she were performing surgery instead of giving a bath. Laughing out loud, she stood on the edge of the bathtub to brace Mrs. Petrocelli as she was lowered into the water by two orderlies. And this was no easy task. Remember, this patient was comatose and wasn't exactly going to hold herself upright.

Well, at this point Toni really sort of became some kind of a surgeon. Ever so slowly and carefully, Toni cut off Mrs. Petrocelli's bun. She held it up. It looked like a shrunken head, with a few hairs sticking straight out. It was solid as a rock, packed with stool and it stunk like crazy. Toni dropped the bun into a waiting garbage bag and somebody took the bag right out of the unit. The operation was a success.

Then Toni bathed Mrs. Petrocelli and washed her short hair. That was quite a team effort, since the patient had to be supported so that she didn't sink under the water. And during all of this, somebody carefully watched Mrs. Petrocelli's respirations and pulse. Remember, she still was an I.C.U. patient. Most unorthodox intensive care, as it was.

Somebody Upstairs must have been watching over Mrs. Petrocelli. With I.V. fluids to hydrate her and tube feedings to nourish her, she soon started to improve. With the combination of antibiotics and skin care, her wounds healed and her skin became soft and smooth. It turned out that Mrs. Petrocelli had naturally curly hair and by the time she had regained consciousness and looked in a mirror, she really liked what she saw. The short curly hair framed her face and made her look a lot younger. Although she certainly must have wondered what happened to her hair, she never asked. And nobody volunteered to tell her what her dog had done.

Mrs. Petrocelli could not go back to living alone, and was discharged to a very nice nursing home. Her dog was adopted by her next door neighbor. And nobody ever officially asked what happened to that bun. But everyone knew that the haircut was a very important part of Mrs. Petrocelli's nursing care that night. And everyone also knows that Toni went over and above the call of duty.

But isn't that what real nurses do?

The Crosstown Bus

It was dinner time and a group of nurses were seated together in the cafeteria, one of the rare opportunities they had to actually leave the floors. It was a mixed crew. Brand new nurses as well as seasoned veterans filled the long table in the rear of the large room.

They always sat in the back, no matter how many empty tables there were close to the door. It was as if the nurses could hide that way, or at least get a break from the frantic pace of the hospital. If nobody could see them, then nobody could bother them.

Well, this particular night, one of the nurses had walked into the co-ed single stall staff bathroom and had found one of the male physicians just getting up off the toilet. She hadn't really seen anything, but both of them were very embarrassed. Everyone was laughing about it and a few of the nurses began to talk about some of their more embarrassing moments.

Wanda was probably the most experienced nurse in the cafeteria that night; in other words, she was the oldest. She had been around hospitals for an awful lot of years and had seen more than many of those nurses combined. But as for her own embarrassing moment, well!!!!!

She had been a junior in nursing school, a very large hospital based school in New York City. It was back in the days when students worked the wards from early morning until late at night and, in fact, were paid a monthly stipend for doing so. There were strict evening curfews and all the girls (and of course they were all girls) had to be back inside by ten o'clock at night. Roll call was at seven a.m. every single morning, and so the students rarely went out after dinner. They were just too tired.

Well, on this particular Friday, Wanda had finished up at around five o'clock, and on the spur of the moment, she decided she was going to go home for the weekend. She had to catch the crosstown bus, switch to the Seventh Avenue subway, and then take the Long Island Railroad from Penn Station. It was July, right in the middle of a New York heat wave, and there was no air conditioning anywhere in the big old hospital buildings. Her clothes were damp with perspiration.

By the time Wanda got back to her room and took off her starched bib and apron, her blue plaid top, and her heavy white nurse's cap, it was rush hour in the Big Apple. Changing into her street clothes, she threw her uniform down the laundry chute, and crammed two weeks worth of dirty underwear into her tiny overnight case. Wanda

28

grabbed her pocketbook and the blue overnight case and flew downstairs to the lobby of the fourteen story student nurses' building.

Knowing she needed to make the six forty-nine out of Penn Station, Wanda had to rush. So she raced to the corner of Fifth Avenue and then over to East Ninety-sixt Street, arriving just in time to see her bus getting ready to leave. Wanda climbed up the steps and dropped her money into the slot. The bus took off.

The bus was totally packed. Solid. Not only were there no seats, but the passengers who were standing were literally pressing against one another. This was no surprising; it was, in fact, a routine rush hour event in New York. And Wanda couldn' even hang on to one of those overhead straps. They were all taken.

Not a problem, she thought. The people were crammed so tightly against each other that there was no way she could fall over. So she stood there as they all did totally ignoring each other. After a few minutes, the bus made a sharp right turn into Central Park and started on the winding road to get through to the west side. It was then that the clasp of her little blue overnight case banged into the handle of an umbrella held by the lady next to her. The pressure of the bang must have hit that clasp just right because in the flash of a second the cover of the hard plastic case flew open and fourteen days of dirty bras, underpants, garter belts and white nylon stockings flew up in the air and onto the laps of the two young men sitting right in front of her.

Well, Wanda was frozen. She was horrified. And she had absolutely no room to move. Even a little bit. Wanda could not bend over to pick up the dirty sweat-dried clothes. She couldn't budge. She was stuck exactly as she was until some of the people got off the bus. Wanda heard herself making little moaning noises. Her face was beet red, and it wasn't from the heat. She just stood there.

The two guys who were now covered with Wanda's smelly clothes were about her age. Wanda, after a quick glance down, couldn't look at them. First she closed her eyes and then she tilted her head back, staring straight up at the roof of the bus, which was still traveling through the park. Wanda was aware, without looking, that the boys were laboriously gathering up her bras and underpants and trying to stuff them back into the overnight case. She felt it more than saw it. Nobody said a word. Nobody at all. There was absolute silence. It was as if the whole front of the bus knew that Wanda was ready to drop dead right there if anyone so much as made a tiny snicker, and it was obvious that she wouldn't even be able to fall to the floor after she died. There was no room.

By the time the bus came out of Central Park and turned onto Seventh Avenue, all of Wanda's underwear had been replaced in her blue overnight case. The young guys had done it, without saying a word. And the clasp had been reclosed. The very first stop was Wanda's, as well as all the people in front of her. Tightly clutching the

29

case with both hands, Wanda climbed down off the bus. She looked at no one and spoke to nobody.

Wanda ran down the steps of the Seventh Avenue subway, and it was only after she pushed through the turnstile that she started to cry. She couldn't believe what had happened. Only nineteen years old, she had been totally mortified. But it was over, and hopefully she would never ever see any of those people again.

Years later, when Wanda could finally tell the story, she was able to laugh at her most embarrassing moment. And, she thought, this really was a tribute to the people of New York City. They say New Yorkers are a tough bunch, but these people instinctively knew what to do. They were really very kind to her. And over the years, when various things happen or she does stupid things, Wanda thinks back to that hot day when she was a nursing student and she publicly lost her underwear. And she doubts that anything will ever top that.

Ready Or Not

Kathy was paged to the ultrasound department. It really didn't seem urgent, and she thought it most likely was to adjust an I.V. or fix a beeping pump. Something routine like that. When she called over there, someone told her that one of the technologists in the back scanning room wanted her to check a patient.

She heard the sound of someone vomiting as she walked toward the rear of the department. And the noise was mixed in with that of water draining into something. Kathy started to run, and as she approached the patient, she saw blood pouring from her mouth. The blood was bubbling out, and as the patient took a breath, she was sucking the blood back in. Into her trachea and down into her lungs. At this point, the lady's eyes were rolled back in her head.

Kathy grabbed a suction set, and, turning the patient's head to the side, she began to try to draw that fresh red blood out of her lungs. The old lady never really stopped breathing, nor did she lose her pulse. Eileen didn't want to call the cardiac arrest code team, because this wasn't a true code. The vital signs were there, but just barely.

Well, Kathy started calling out for equipment and supplies, and the STAT pages called for all the right people. This lady had come down for a quick carotid doppler study, and she had been awake and alert when she initially arrived in the department. By the time she reached the cardiac care unit however, she had a couple of I.V. lines in place, a foley catheter, and was intubated and on a ventilator. Twenty minutes after that, she was on all kinds of drips and had a pulmonary artery catheter in place. By that time, she was as close to death as a person could actually get without crossing over that line. The nurses expected her to die that night.

But she didn't. The next day, Kathy went up to see the lady. She had more or less stabilized, but still was in a coma. Nobody really thought she would live, as she now had a whopping aspiration pneumonia. After all, fresh warm blood doesn't exactly belong in the air spaces of the lungs. But the lady hung on, and before the day had passed, she began to wake up. Her blood pressure had returned to normal and they started to wean her off her drugs.

By the next day, the old lady had really begun to improve, and there was no stopping her. In fact, before long she was taken off the respirator and all her tubes were removed. She felt fine and looked terrific. The lady remembered nothing of what had happened, which was a really good thing, the nurses said. She thought she had simply fainted, which was what had brought her to the hospital in the first place. So she was transferred to a regular room, and soon she was up and about. All her tests had come back normal, and nobody really knew why she had vomited that blood in the first place. They guessed it was from an ulcer caused by all the aspirin she had been taken for her arthritis before she had come to the hospital.

Meanwhile, the lady was fine. And she wanted to go home. So her doctor went in to speak to her, telling her that he would definitely discharge her after a couple of more tests were done to check on that probable ulcer, but other than that she seemed to be quite healthy. She could plan on going home the day after tomorrow, he told her.

The doctor came out to the nurses' station and began to write in her chart. The floor nurse went into the room to do something, and suddenly she yelled for the doctor. It seems the little old lady was dead. No pulse, no breathing, no blood pressure. She was blue and dead. Just like that. Two minutes after the doctor walked out.

So of course they called a code and naturally they worked like crazy. But she was dead. And nothing and nobody could bring her back. Weird. With her doctor, who happened to be a cardiologist, and all the nurses right there when it happened. Well, everyone felt terrible. The lady had been brought back from the brink of death once and had done so well. What had happened was anyone's guess. Maybe the fainting spells she had suffered in the past were related. Maybe it was a heart attack. Or maybe it had just been her time to go, and these past few days had simply been a gift. It depends on what you believe.

The Work Boot

Nobody knew exactly why or how it happened, but just that it did happen. Jerry's crane had somehow touched a high tension wire, and the electricity had come right through the roof of his cab. It had entered his body through the top of his head and traveled down, exiting through his right foot which was touching the brake pedal.

When Jerry was pulled from the crane, he was right in the middle of a grand mal seizure. When the seizure stopped, so did Jerry's breathing. But miraculously, Jerry was resuscitated and he was conscious when he reached the emergency room. The only visible sign of injury was to his scalp. It had been burned away.

In the emergency room Jerry's head wound was treated. His heart was doing funny little things, which was not unexpected since the electrical charge had obviously passed right through it. He was given drugs to stabilize him and he seemed to be settling down. He had an intravenous drip running and was on some nasal oxygen. Jerry still had most of his clothes on, since only his shirt had been removed to attach the leads for the cardiac monitor.

Now it was time to undress Jerry and get him into a gown. He was wearing a pair of heavy jeans and workboots. The nurse, Clair, first removed Jerry's left boot and gray sock. The right boot was a little harder to remove for some reason. She opened the laces a bit more and pulled harder on the boot. It finally started to slide off. Clair tugged harder. There. It was coming off. Holding the heavy boot with both hands, Clair gave one last pull. The boot came loose and she pulled it out of the cuff of the pants. Sticking straight up out of the top of the workboot was Jerry's lower leg, burned right in half. The two long bones, with their black charred tops, extended about eight inches further than the top of the boot.

Clair was totally horrified. As an experienced emergency room nurse, she had seen a lot. But this was something else. It was as if Clair had pulled off Jerry's leg. That's the feeling she got. But the worst thing about this was that Jerry, who had no sensation in his leg, witnessed the whole thing. It was unbelievable. Jerry started to scream out loud. It was a nightmare for everybody. They had to hold Jerry down and cut off his pants at the same time, knowing that they were going to find the upper ends of his tibia and fibula sticking out. And there they were.

After a lot of sedation, Jerry finally fell asleep. Clair was still a wreck and could hardly function. Jerry was put on call for the operating room to have his scalp debrided

33

and his leg wound fixed up. He was considered a very sick young man, since electrical burns do a lot more damage than just what is obvious. Kidney failure, infection, and shock were just some of what could lie ahead for him.

Well, since Jerry was going to be sent directly from the operating room to what was known as the Surgical I.C.U./Recovery Room, his papers and personal belongings were sent up ahead of him. Everything was delivered to the reception area of this big twenty-two bed unit, where it was the ward clerk's responsibility to log all the items in.

The place was wild that afternoon. It was short staffed and crowded with people, with all the problems happening at once, a scene not unusual for an I.C.U. in a big county hospital. So there was confusion and noise and phones ringing and patients calling and everything else going on. Trudy, the ward clerk, had just come on duty and was trying to clear up the big mess on her desk. One of the first orders of business was to get the belongings checked in and put away. That would, at least, make the place appear a little neater.

Patients' personal effects were delivered to the floors in big brown paper bags and at this time there were two bags on the desk. Trudy took care of the first one, separating and recording its contents. Then it was time for Jerry's stuff. His bag was heavy. Trudy looked inside and saw a brown workboot right on top. That's why the bag weighed so much, she thought. Those big boots were really something. Trudy dumped the bag upside down on the desk. There was one boot, a shirt and a wristwatch. There were more things in the bag, but they were jammed in there. Stuck.

Trudy put her hand in the bag and pulled at the top of an undershirt. But something was caught in the shirt and it wouldn't come loose. Trudy gave a yank and everything tumbled onto the desk. And there, right in the middle, was that right boot with the foot sticking out.

Trudy didn't say a word. Her face drained of all its color, she projectile vomited, and then passed out right there on the floor. Some moron in the E.R. had put the boot with the foot in the bag with all Jerry's clothes. It was like something from a horror film. Poor Trudy. She was, to begin with, one of those people who worked in hospitals but who could never stand to hear about or see anything yucky. Of all people to have this happen to.

Well, Trudy went home shortly after this unfortunate event. She was physically sick from what she saw. She stayed out for two days, and when she came back she warned everyone to say absolutely nothing about what had happened. Nobody ever mentioned it to her. Jerry's hospital course was not smooth. He developed lots of complications and problems and needed three months to progress enough to be sent to a rehabilitation facility.

As for poor Trudy, a month to the day after the boot fiasco, she was brought into the same emergency room with a subarachnoid hemorrhage. She died the next day, and some people said that maybe the stress of what happened to her caused the wall of the aneurysm which she never knew she had to get weaker. Not likely, but then, who really knows for sure?

Dopey Things Smart Nurses Do

1. Valium broke the seizure easily. Linda's patient was now sleeping quietly, obviously in the post-ictal stage. Linda took the now empty syringe and re-capped it. She stuck it in her right uniform pocket, sharp end down, in order to dispose of it later in the medication room. However, there was one minor problem. As the syringe was entering Linda's pocket, the plastic cap flew off and she stuck the needle, all one and a half inches of it, right through the cotton uniform pocket directly into her abdomen.

Even though all she got from this was a black and blue mark on her belly, Linda was certain that she had at least punctured an organ or two.

2. Lori was just about to give her patient an I.M. injection. She grasped the patient's muscle with the fingers of her left hand and, with her right, wiped the area with alcohol. Then, as too many nurses do, Lori picked up the syringe and moved it toward her mouth. She had all the intentions of popping off the plastic cap which covered the needle with her teeth, as she had done hundreds of times before. However, this time the cap had already popped off, and Lori plunged the long 22 gauge needle, all the way up to the hub, into the roof of her mouth.

Lori was absolutely certain that her brain was going to herniate down into her mouth and kill her. Obviously, it didn't.

(These two events happened way before the A.I.D.S. epidemic and the onset of needle precautions!!!)

3. The patient was known to have tremendous esophageal varices, grossly distended varicose veins in the top of the stomach and the esophagus. As every nurse knows, these large veins are formed from the greatly elevated pressures which back up from the compromised circulation to the liver. And as every nurse certainly should know, these varices are large and, because of the increased pressures, they can rupture and result in massive bleeding. Well, one night this patient suffered a cardio-pulmonary arrest. Ellen, after calling the cardiac arrest code, prepared to do CPR. Instead of grabbing the Ambu bag which was just down the hall, Ellen began to do mouth to mouth. The force from the chest compressions which were being performed by another

36

nurse obviously exploded one of the varices, since almost instantly great gobs of blood burst forth from the patient's mouth and spewed into Ellen's.

4. Marie had just applied an inch of nitrobid ointment to the patient's upper chest. She put the tube down and washed her hands at the sink in his room. Then she returned to the bedside to speak to the patient. Marie stood there, chattering away to him. Boy, were her hands dry, she thought absentmindedly. All that handwashing that nurses do really dries out the skin. Without thinking, Marie idly coated her hands with some lotion and rubbed it in. Still jabbering to the patient, she massaged the lotion into all the cracks and crevices of both hands. The lotion really felt soothing. Then Marie looked down. Instead of applying the Keri lotion, she had done the job with the nitrobid cream. About half of the tube. Marie ran to the sink and soaped up her hands and washed the stuff off.

Although certain she was going to get a horrible headache and dilate all her blood vessels and drop her blood pressure to zero and die, not a thing happened.

5. And speaking of nitrobid - - - Carol's patient had multiple small ulcers in the mucus membranes of her nose. She was supposed to have some type of topical cream applied four times a day. It came in a little tube and the nurses squirted the stuff on an applicator and then stuck the applicator in her nostrils to coat the mucus membranes. So that's exactly what Carol did. However, instead of the medication ordered especially for the ulcers, Carol coated this lady's nasal membranes with nitrobid ointment. And, as we all know, medication is absorbed very rapidly through mucus membranes. So Carol, once she realized what she had done, was sure the lady was going to die. Naturally, she went nuts, trying to wipe the ointment off, but simply rubbed it in deeper.

However, besides a very slight drop in blood pressure, nothing at all happened. If the patient got a terrible headache, nobody knew about it. She was already comatose.

6. Diane's patient had suffered a massive nosebleed, so severe that the usual nasal packing didn't work. He needed to have a foley catheter inserted into his nose and the catheter balloon inflated with saline to provide continuous pressure against the bleeding vessels. It seemed to have worked. The bleeding had slowed to a trickle, and then stopped. The patient, who had been quite confused before all this happened, was very sick. He had lots of lines and tubes. So it was early morning, at the change of shift. Diane, a brand new nurse, was giving report to the day staff. She noted that the patient had an order to remove the foley catheter that day. And Diane, always helpful, told the day nurse that she had already taken out the foley. The day nurse had a funny feeling. "Diane," she said, choosing her words carefully. "You did take out the foley in

37

is bladder, didn't you? His urinary foley." Diane became pale. "Oh, my God," she said quietly. "I probably killed him."

Well, Diane didn't kill her patient. He didn't bleed to death. It was just about time for the catheter in his nose to come out anyway. And Diane's fledgling career as a nurse was not over, as she most definitely thought. The doctor didn't hate her and she wasn't fired.

A Slice of the Pie

It was time for her to leave for the day, but she still had one person scheduled for a scan. The working diagnosis was "rule out aortic dissection". Nobody really believed that diagnosis for a 30 year old. The young man, Alan, had been sitting at his desk at work when he began to have chest pains, which "went straight through to my back." he walked into his physician's office looking pretty healthy. But just to be safe, the physician had sent him for the computerized tomography (CT) scan. And of course, he had driven himself to the hospital. Why not?

By the time Alan was ready to be scanned he still looked good, and he said he really didn't feel sick. If it wasn't for the fact that his father had some kind of unexplained sudden death at the age of thirty-one, he really would have ignored the pain. But the CT scan revealed that Alan had a huge aneurysm in his thoracic aorta that was getting ready to rupture. If it did, Alan would join his father in heaven, who probably had gotten there due to the same thing.

Alan's physician arrived in the hospital just as the radiologist had finished reading the films and was frantically trying to reach him. Judy, the radiology nurse, had run to get a stretcher. As the two physicians and Judy brought the stretcher to the doorway of the large waiting room, they found Alan sitting in the corner, idly thumbing through a magazine.

His physician walked in, took him by the hand, and helped him get on the stretcher. "We're going to the emergency room. I'll explain as we go," he told Alan. "You are a very sick man." Alan looked stunned as the trio pushed the stretcher down the hall to the emergency department. Alan's physician, as gently as he could, explained that the major artery in his body was beginning to leak, and the only way to keep it from bursting and killing him was to open his chest and fix the leak immediately.

But the aneurysm was high up in the chest and Alan would need to be on cardiopulmonary bypass while his heart was stopped and the leak repaired. Since the small community hospital was not equipped for this surgery, Alan needed to be transferred right way. So Judy, who had met Alan just a short while ago, became his substitute family as well as his nurse. In between attaching the cardiac leads and starting an I.V., Judy held Alan's hand and reassured him. Terrified, he hung on to her as if she were his lifeline. Within a few minutes, Alan was sped away in an ambulance.

Two minutes later Alan's wife arrived in the emergency room department completely hysterical. Judy and the physician took her into a conference room and explained everything. Judy stayed with her until her parents arrived to drive with her to the other hospital. Only then did Judy leave the E.D. and return to radiology. The next morning, Judy arrived at work early. She hadn't slept very well, knowing just how high the mortality rate really was for a dissecting aortic aneurysm. But she received terrific news: Alan had made it into the operating before the aneurysm blew. And he had sailed through the operation without any major complications. Alan was fine and was expected to make a complete recovery.

Three weeks later, Alan arrived in the emergency department carrying two pies. One was for the ER nurses and one was for Judy. He told her that he didn't remember much about that afternoon because everything had happened too fast. But he mostly remembered Judy and the fact that she was there for him -- she was his strength.

Later on, after Alan had gone, everyone wondered about the pies. Lots of people bring cakes or cookies or buns or even flowers. But why did he buy a pie? Maybe it was a "guy" thing. But maybe not. Somebody had a thought that maybe, without realizing it, Alan chose the pies as symbols of how many people it took to save his life. And each, in a special way, contributed a small slice of the pie to make Alan whole and healthy again.

"A Slice of the Pie" by Linda Strangio RN, MA, CCRN. From: *The Nursing Spectrum*, New York/New Jersey Metro Edition. Reprinted with permission.

Visiting Hours

It was visiting hours and the little old lady had come to see her husband. The man had suffered a stroke three days earlier, but was now progressing nicely.

The CT Scan department had called for the patient to come down for a routine follow-up scan, and so he had been taken downstairs. The man's wife, since she had a little trouble walking, decided that she would wait in his room instead of accompanying him to the radiology department. He wouldn't be gone very long, the nurses told her.

So the little old lady was sitting quietly in a chair next to the bed, looking at the television. Being a hot day, she had come to the hospital dressed only in a thin cotton housecoat. On her feet were a pair of shoes which looked a lot like slippers, the kind you stick your feet into and just shuffle around in. The room was quiet, except for the low drone of the T.V. The lady wasn't bothering anyone, just sitting there watching the afternoon soaps.

After a few minutes, in strode two orderlies. These guys were terrific. Besides needing very little direction and doing whatever needed to be done, they were fast and efficient and extremely kind to everyone. Now it was the middle of the afternoon, and they had been called to help get some of the patients back to bed. The nurses were all still in report, but these orderlies were perfectly capable of making what they called, "Back To Bed Rounds." Alone. Without any help from the nursing staff.

"Time to go back to bed, Ma'am," cheerily announced Henry, popping his head into the man's room. "I guess you've been up a while. You must be getting tired." The little old lady was confused. "I don't want to go to bed," she protested softly. "I'm just waiting for my husband." Henry smiled. "You can wait for him in bed," he answered with his usual big grin.

Now the lady started to become uneasy. What did this man mean that she could wait for him in bed? Just what kind of hanky panky did he think was going on anyway? What kind of a place was this? Before she could say another word, Henry bent down and pulled off her slipper-like shoes. "Come on, Ma'am," he said pleasantly. "You're so little that I will just pick you up and put you in bed." And Henry scooped the little old lady up in his strong arms and deposited her gently right in the middle of her husband's freshly made bed. "There you are," Henry announced. "Nice and comfy in your pretty little nightgown." He pulled the crisp white sheet up over the little lady and turned to leave the room. "Someone will be here shortly," he said with a wink.

41

The little old lady started to scream. She had no clue what was going on, only that some crazy man had thrown her into bed, insinuating that something was going to happen to her soon. Unable to put down the siderails, she was a wild woman by the time one of the nurses came in. And since this was the very beginning of the shift, that nurse hadn't yet seen all of the twelve patients assigned to her. So all she knew was that she had a confused little old lady who was dressed in a bright floral nightgown and was sitting bolt upright in her bed, screaming like a maniac.

The nurse, as much as she tried, could not get this lady to stop screaming. She looked terrified. So the nurse went out to check the Cardex to see if the lady had anything ordered for sedation. Hey, wait a minute, the nurse said to herself. According to her records, there should be a man in that bed. So who was the lady?

Well, to make a long story short, they finally realized what had happened. The lady was helped out of bed and finally, after what seemed like an eternity, she calmed down. Everyone explained and apologized again and again, but nobody was really sure that the lady really understood why the mistake was made. Or, for that matter, that it really was a mistake.

Until the time of his discharge, the patient's wife never sat down in his room again. She stood at what looked to be rigid attention, with her pocketbook clutched in front of her at all times. She seemed to be waiting for some lunatic to come in and grab her or something. Visiting hours were not exactly happy hours.

The Shower

No wonder he was scared. He was only twenty-seven years old and he was hurt and far from home.

John had been in an auto accident just a few hours earlier. New to his company, he had been on his way home from a seminar when his car skidded off the road. Although the car was badly damaged, it still could be driven. Along with the multiple lacerations and bruises on his face, the side of his chest had hit the steering wheel or dashboard. John knew he was hurt, but he refused to get into the ambulance which had been called by the police. John did, however, agree to drive himself to the emergency room of the local hospital there.

The emergency department was very quiet when John arrived. He parked his damaged car in the lot and walked up the ramp. John noticed that his right side hurt when he breathed and he was only able to take short rapid breaths. The triage nurse took John directly into an examining room, and when John took off his blood stained shirt, a small bruise could be seen on his right upper chest area.

John had a chest x-ray taken and after just a few minutes, the emergency room doctor informed him that besides suffering two broken ribs, about seventy per-cent of John's right lung had collapsed. He needed to have a tube inserted right away in order for the lung to re-expand.

Wait a minute, John told the emergency room staff. Nobody was going to put anything into his chest, unless he could drive himself home with it. You see, he told them, he sure wasn't staying in that hospital. As kind and efficient as they all were, he was going home. If he really had to be in a hospital, it would be the one near his home, and where his own doctor worked.

John was crazy, the staff told him. How did he think he was going to get home? Why, he was going to drive his car, he answered. It may have been damaged, but it was alright to drive. No way, the nurses and doctors said. His lung had collapsed and at any time, he could get into real trouble. His heart and the left lung could shift over toward the right side, and that could become a life threatening emergency. He couldn't do it. John smiled. Oh, yes he could, he answered quietly. He would drive directly to the hospital near his house, the one in which he had his appendix removed two years earlier, and the one which took care of his father when he had suffered a heart attack. He was going home.

So John signed the paper that showed he was leaving against medical advice. The doctor wrote an addendum on the bottom of the form, which explained that John had been told the seriousness of his situation and had still insisted on leaving. John thanked the staff for their concern, and he promised he would somehow get word to them later that night that he was alright. But he was leaving.

Holding the palm of his left hand against the broken ribs on the right side, John slowly walked out of the door, down the ramp, and out to the parking lot. He knew he'd make it.

Just under two hours later, John pulled up outside the hospital near his home. The sun had set and it was getting cold and windy. By this time John had really become short of breath. He was exhausted and his whole body ached. But he was there. He was home.

The emergency department receptionist was expecting John. The transferring physician had already called John's doctor, who, in turn, had notified the emergency room that this young guy with a seventy percent pneumothorax would be arriving. It was obvious that most of the staff thought John was a little nuts to drive more than fifty miles with a collapsed lung, but they also understood why he did it. After all, nobody wants to be away from home in a strange place when they are sick or hurt.

Well, apparently John had been booked into the intensive care unit, and he was to be a direct admission there. He had brought his x-rays with him and a chest surgeon was going to meet him there to put in his chest tube. So they put John on a stretcher and wheeled him up to the I.C. U. where John's bed was waiting.

Gina was John's nurse that night when he first arrived in the unit. John was dirty and sweaty and his hair was matted with dried blood. His clothes were muddy from where he had lain on the wet grass after the accident, and they too were blood streaked. His entire body was covered with grime. John was a mess. He looked miserable and uncomfortable. Gina wheeled John into the room where the I.C.U. bed stood waiting, made up with fresh clean linen. The I.V. set-up was ready, as was the nasal oxygen. Gina looked at the bed and then looked at John. She could just imagine how he felt. Gina hesitated as an idea popped into her head.

John had driven his car for two hours and had made it without any tragedies happening. Surely he could last another five minutes. "John," Gina said quietly. "How would you like to take a nice hot shower?" John smiled at Gina, his eyes opening wide. He just nodded, probably imagining how good that would feel.

Without another word Gina turned and wheeled the stretcher back out of the room, into the center of the unit. She went over to the linen cart and pulled off a clean gown and a couple of towels. She stopped in the clean utility room and grabbed a bar of Dial and a small packet of castile enema soap. Gina piled the stuff on the stretcher nd continued on out of the unit to the elevators. She told the other nurses to say John adn't arrived yet if his doctors or anyone else came for him.

Gina pushed the stretcher onto the elevator and took it to the fourth floor. They ot off and Gina wheeled John into the closest general medical-surgical floor corridor. There were three bathrooms at the end of the hall, one of which had a stall shower. The all was empty. "O.K., John," Gina said quietly. "This is it. Get off this stretcher, and ake the fastest shower you ever took. I'll wait outside, and don't you dare faint or nything in there. And, handing him the packet of enema soap, she added, "Here's your hampoo." John took the soap with the words "for soap suds enemas" on the package nd smiled. "Don't worry," he answered, all the while taking tiny little painful breaths. 'I'll be fine."

Five minutes later John came out of the bathroom. His hair was dripping and ome of his cuts and abrasions were oozing a little blood. But he looked like he felt a ot better, and he smelled good, like Dial soap. Gina had put a clean sheet on the stretcher and John painfully climbed up and lay down. Gina covered him with a blanket nd off they went, back to the I.C.U. Nobody on the fourth floor had paid a bit of attention to either of them. As they wheeled through the doors of the intensive care unit, one of the other nurses asked where they had gone. "To take a shower," Gina answered simply. Nobody even questioned it.

Well, by the time the shift had ended, John had his chest tube inserted and hooked up to suction. His right lung had already expanded and he was able to breathe normally. He had his I.V. in place and he was receiving antibiotics. He was on oxygen and attached to a pulse oximeter. Demerol had taken away the pain so that he could relax and visit with his family. And he was already getting better.

The next day, John left the I.C.U. and was transferred to a regular floor. Before he was discharged, he stopped down in the unit to say goodbye to Gina. He told her that he knew what a big risk she had taken, sneaking him up to take a shower. Of all the treatments and medication he received, he said, that hot shower was the thing that helped the most. "Thank you," John told her. "You made the difference."

Nurse Abuse

1. George Smith seemed to be improving. He had come through raging D.T.'s and was now much quieter. Still loosely restrained, Mr. Smith was lying quietly in bed. His yelling had stopped, and it appeared that he no longer was hallucinating. Bob was kneeling at the side of Mr. Smith's bed, draining the foley bag into a plastic graduate, when the man suddenly sat bolt upright. Without a second's warning, Mr. Smith pulled his arms loose from the wrist bands, reached over the side rail, and got both hands around Bob's neck. Then squeezing as hard as he could, Mr. Smith proceeded to fracture Bob's larynx.

2. It was a little after six o'clock and Eileen was passing out her six o'clock medications. She entered Mrs. McLaughlin's room with a small plastic cup filled with some pills. "Here's your medicine," cheerily announced Eileen. "Get out," responded Mrs. McLaughlin. "I don't want any pills. I'm trying to take a nap." Eileen bent over the bed. "Come on, Mrs. McLaughlin," she persuaded. "Take the medicine and I'll leave so you can sleep." Mrs. McLaughlin slowly pulled herself up in bed. "Give me the cup," she said. Eileen held the small plastic cup out toward the lady's outstretched hand. Mrs. McLaughlin grabbed the cup and threw the pills right into Eileen's face. Then, before Eileen could even react, Mrs. McLaughlin grabbed Eileen's hand and with both of hers, she bent back Eileen's thumb until it dislocated.

3. Diane was out in the hall with Mr. Fendy, trying to get him to ambulate. Mr. Fendy, a big strong man, had just undergone major abdominal surgery and really needed to get moving. He didn't want to do anything but stay in bed, saying that walking hurt too much. "I want to go back to bed," whined Mr. Fendy. "It hurts to walk." Diane nodded. "I know it hurts, Mr. Fendy," she answered. "But walking and exercising is good for you and it will help you recover faster." Mr. Fendy stopped short. "You want to see me exercise?" asked Mr. Fendy with a weird look on his face. "How's this for exercise?" With that the man drew back his arm, and with his hand clenched in a tight fist, soundly punched Diane right in the jaw.

4. Miss Bartch had been admitted with a spontaneous pneumothorax, and the tube which had been put into her chest was helping her lung to expand. Naturally, it

46

hurt a little bit, and even more so when she coughed and took deep breaths. Marlene was Miss Bartch's nurse and she noticed that her breathing sounded a bit moist and crackly. Concerned that the patient might be getting a bit congested, Marlene spent a little time trying to get the lady to cough up some of the junk in her lungs. "Come on, Miss Bartch," urged Marlene. "Cough up that stuff." Then attempting to support the sore area around the tube, Marlene pressed both her hands against the dressing. "Now cough," she said. "You're killing me," screamed Miss Bartch. Then, with no warning she drew back her right leg, and with all her strength, kicked Marlene right in the center of her abdomen. Marlene went flying across the room, and then doubled up on the floor.

5. Mrs. Hanley was a sweet little old lady. Mildly confused, she was basically a cooperative patient who could easily be reoriented to her surroundings. Lauren had just given Mrs. Hanley a bedbath, and now was trying to clean the crusts off her dry lips. With what seemed to be the speed of light, the little lady lunged forward with her head, and then bit down as hard as she could on Lauren's hand. Her teeth went right down to the bone and stayed there. It took a lot of effort to pry Mrs. Hanley loose, and by that time, Lauren had literally passed out from the shock of what had happened.

Are these rare events? They most certainly are not, and by some standards, these are quite mild. Ask any E.R. or psych nurse.

A Change of Pace

He had been admitted earlier on the day shift with some bogus diagnosis like change in mental status." His regular doctor was away, and the covering physician was the one who had put James in the hospital solely on the basis of the history given by the family.

James was in perpetual motion. He jogged up and down the unit, at the speed of whirlwind. He wouldn't or couldn't sit still, and it was obvious to everyone that he didn't belong on a general medical-surgical floor. In today's times, James never would have been admitted, but this is now and that was then.

So there was James, parked in room 618. There was no psychiatric unit back then. He disrupted the whole floor with his antics. One of the nurses had overheard his sister talking to their brother, whispering that they deserved this "break" from James, and how it was "someone else's turn to put up with him." So the staff guessed that this really was not a change in mental status at all, but simply a way to get rid of him for a while.

The only orders the nurses had for James was to "observe" him. How could anybody not observe James? He walked in and out of the nurses' station and in big circles from the clean utility room, through the report room, and back to the dirty utility room. And then he did it again. And again. And again.

When he got tired of that, he came to the nurses' station and asked questions like, "What are you doing? Who are you talking to on the phone? Why is that man on a stretcher? What's in that drawer?" And so on. The nurses didn't know what to do.

At seven o'clock, James was back at the desk. "Could I have a razor?" he asked. "I really need a shave." Joan, who knew James wasn't suicidal (just nuts) gave him a razor to shut him up. The next time James swung by the nurses station on his race around the unit, he was bald as a billiard ball. "I told you I needed a shave," he smiled. "Doesn't that look better?" Joan just groaned, the only thing on her mind by now being whether or not she now needed to fill out an incident report.

By eight o'clock, the nurses were ready to scream. James was in the back report room, rifling through the lab coats hanging on the hooks. "I need a change of clothes," James cheerily called out. "Don't worry. I don't need any help. I'll find something here." Nobody cared. They just wanted him to shut up. If wearing a lab coat could make him happy, then let him wear a lab coat.

A few minutes later Dr. Pincus entered the unit. He was an attendin
nephrologist and he had his wife with him. They were on their way out to dinner. D
Pincus introduced his wife to the nurses and then led her into the report room, askin
her to stay there and wait for him while he saw his patients. Mrs. Pincus sat down an
started to read a magazine.

At that minute, James emerged from his room and strode past the nurses' statio
He was wearing the lab coat, but as he zipped around the corner, it quickly becam
apparent to Joan that the lab coat was all he was wearing. Except for a bunch of pen
he had stuffed in the breast pocket, James was naked as a jay bird.

Before Joan could say anything, James entered the report room and flew over t
Dr. Pincus' wife. James plopped himself into the chair next to her and started to jabbe
non-stop. Joan couldn't hear anything he was saying, but she noted that Mrs. Pincu
seemed to be a little bewildered. And Mrs. Pincus obviously had not looked at the fror
of the unbuttoned lab coat either. As Joan was about to go in to "rescue" the poo
woman, Dr. Pincus appeared in the nurses' station to ask for a chart. "Oh," he saic
smiling. "I see my wife has someone to keep her company."

"Uh, duhh, Dr. Pincus," mumbled Joan idiotically. "I think you should know tha
the man sitting next to your wife is not one of the residents. He actually is a psyc
patient and he is totally naked under that lab coat." And then Joan giggled nervously.

Dr. Pincus did not giggle back. He obviously didn't think anything was funny.
"Maria," he bellowed at his wife. "Come out here right now!" Maria jumped up anc
ran out of the report room. Dr. Pincus threw the chart that he was holding back on the
desk, grabbed Maria's arm and pulled her out of the unit. He never looked back. Bu
Maria did, just in time to see James come whizzing around the corner with his open lat
coat flying in the breeze. And it was clear that this time she did look down, because he
eyes and her mouth flew open with a silent scream. And then they were gone. Tha
dinner party they were off to is going to have some lively conversation, Joan thought.

So what happened to James? Absolutely nothing. He spent the night in the uni
and the next day his own doctor came in and discharged James back to the care of the
family. Except for the fact that James was now bald, their home lives went on as
before. The unit got quiet again, at least back to the way it usually was. A few days
later, when Joan tried to explain things to Dr. Pincus, he simply told her that he didn'
want to hear and he didn't want to know. Let it be, he said. It's better that way.

Dracula

They were pouring meds together and joking about last night. Now that it was over, Cathy could laugh. It wasn't funny, though, at the time.

It seems that Cathy's son, Corey, had gone to his room and was lying on his bed reading a book. Suddenly Corey had called out to his mother that there was a bird flying around his window. When Cathy had come in to investigate, she found the bird was flying around the window, all right, but inside the room. And it wasn't a bird, but a bat.

Cathy had gone nuts, screaming and yelling and scaring the poor kid out of his mind. They both had run out of the room like wild maniacs, and vowed never to return until the bat was gone. Well, Cathy's husband was immediately made the bat hunter, and he chased the little thing all around the house with a mop. Cathy and Corey hid downstairs while the crazed bat hunt took place, and after almost an hour, Cathy's husband was sure he had trapped the bat in the spare room on the third floor. By this time the poor man was totally exhausted, and he announced he was quitting the bat business for the day. He was going to bed. The bat could wait till the next day, since it was safely snared upstairs away from all of them.

Well, Cathy couldn't sleep. She was sure that the bat was going to somehow sneak out of that room and attack them while they slept, so she decided she was going to sleep in the bed with her son in order to protect him if the bat should return. So Cathy got into the bed with Corey, who by this time, was fast asleep. Cathy's husband was also in a deep sleep; that she could tell by the loud snores coming from the master bedroom.

Cathy was wide awake. She gave up trying to sleep, and decided she was just going to lie in the bed and wait until it was time to get up to go to work. She was too wound up. Well, within twenty minutes, Cathy heard a sound at the window. It was the same window where they first had found the bat. At first Cathy was sure she was imagining things. Her nerves were on edge. But what was that shadow behind the window shade? The streetlight in front of the house was reflecting off the window and there was something there.

Suddenly Cathy saw it. It was the bat. It was back. It probably had never gone up to the third floor room after all; Cathy's husband had just told her that to shut her up so they could all get some sleep. Cathy went berserk. She started to scream for her husband in the next room. However, due to the fact that she had the covers pulled up over her and Corey's head, her screams came out muffled and far away. And add that to the sound of a freight train frequency of snoring, there was no way she could be heard.

By this time, Corey was crying and Cathy was too. Checking to make sure the bat was still at the window, Cathy and Corey threw off the covers and bolted from the bed. They ran out of the room and slammed the door behind them. That was it. The screaming and yelling started up again, and Cathy's husband knew he had to get that bat.

Well, a little while later it was all over. The bat was dead and flushed down the toilet. It took a few more hours until the household could finally get to sleep, but finally they did. And at six o'clock in the morning, everyone was up again, getting dressed to start the day. Nice restful night.

So anyway, Cathy and Charlene were in the medication room, going over the events of the evening and laughing out loud. It was over now. Charlene finished what she was doing and decided to take a walk to the pharmacy to pick up a couple of drugs that were missing from her bins. She wanted to start passing her meds, and it was quicker than waiting for the next pharmacy delivery.

Charlene walked out of her unit and down the hall. She turned the corner and cut through the corridor which connected her building to the next, the one in which the pharmacy was housed. As she left her building, she noticed that the big fire doors were closed. That was funny, thought Charlene. She hadn't heard any fire bells or any announcement about a fire drill.

Charlene slowly pushed open the doors. The first thing she noticed were three or four maintenance men standing around. There were ladders and tools on the ground, but the men were just huddled in a group. They seemed to be looking at something on the floor. "Is something wrong?" asked Charlene. One of the men stepped back and pointed to a spot in the corner. Charlene stepped closer to get a good look. She couldn't believe her eyes. There on the floor was a bat. It was covered with blood, red bat blood, and its wings were twitching.

Without a word, Charlene turned and ran back the way she had come. Her eyes wide and wild, she flew into her unit, almost banging into Cathy who was just coming out of the medication room. Charlene could hardly speak. "A bat! A bat! There's a bat by the pharmacy," she finally spit out. "Come with me!" Cathy got pale. She just shook her head. "No, no," she whimpered. I don't want to see another bat. I can't."

Charlene understood. But she was like a woman possessed. She had to see what was going on. Maybe the bats are taking over the world, she thought to herself, on the verge of hysteria. Charlene slowed her steps when she got back to that corridor where the buildings merged. This time the fire doors were open. Charlene tiptoed

51

own the hall, scarcely breathing. She half expected to find that a clan of vampire bats ad commandeered the building or something. Instead, she found nobody there. Maybe the maintenance men were eaten up or taken away by the herd of bats, Charlene nought to herself, and then she found herself laughing out loud at how crazy she was cting. But it was a shrill, panicky laugh.

The only thing in that corridor was a styrofoam coffee cup, on the floor in the orner. And stuffed in that cup was the dead bat. It looked so tiny with its wings folded p, smaller than an egg. Obviously, one of the workmen had put it in the cup and then ney had left. Charlene noticed then that one of the ceiling tiles had been removed and it vas on the floor next to a ladder. Obviously, the bat had come from there. So much for er theory of a mad herd of vampire bats.

Well, Charlene and Cathy finally calmed down enough to call the housekeeping ffice to tell them what had happened. The lady who answered the phone didn't seem at ll excited; she just said that someone would get there soon to take the cup away. Charlene went back to "bat patrol", figuring it was her sworn duty to warn people about he dead bat. She soon realized nobody had the foggiest idea what was in the coffee up; people were just sauntering down the hall and taking care of whatever business hey needed to do. Nobody even glanced at the bat filled cup, and the few people to vhom Charlene showed it really didn't seem all that excited. It was not a very big deal.

Well, Cathy never found another bat in her house, and over the years Charlene never heard any more stories about bats loose in the hospital. Either that was the only ittle bat who had somehow flown in from up in the ceiling, or the total society of nurse-ating vampire bats which had purposely inhabited their hospital decided to move on.

She'd never know for sure.

Life After Death

It started with a vague feeling of indigestion, almost as soon as he awakened that morning. He'd had it before, once or twice, but never like this. He took some Tums, expecting the burning to go away, but it didn't.

Maybe after he ate something he would feel better, he guessed. But nothing changed, and now the burning seemed to have changed to more of a pressure feeling. Taking two more Tums, he sat down in a chair by the front door. He didn't feel right, and now he was beginning to perspire. His left shoulder hurt, too.

Frank's wife knew something was wrong right away. Over his objections, Suzanne called their doctor, who told her to bring him directly to the emergency room. Even though Frank was only thirty-two years old and it was highly unlikely, it could be his heart, he said. Frank needed to be seen right away. So Suzanne packed up their three kids and got them into the car. Frank, naturally, wanted to drive, but Suzanne wouldn't hear of it.

Dropping him off at the emergency room door, Suzanne left with the kids to park the car. As she pulled away, she caught a glimpse of Frank as he walked through the big double doors. Frank was moving very slowly, with his right hand over the center of the chest. Suzanne shuddered. She had a sudden chill.

Not five minutes later, Suzanne arrived with the kids in tow. They were two, four, and five years old. As soon as she neared the emergency room main desk, a nurse came out to meet her. "Are you Mrs. Tomaso?" she asked. When Suzanne nodded, the nurse, Irene, escorted her down the hall into an empty room. "Your husband is very sick, Mrs. Tomaso," Irene said gently. "It's his heart." As Suzanne sat there, frozen in fear, she heard numerous STAT calls for help. E.K.G., respiratory, anesthesia - - people were flying in and out of some room around the corner. There was no doubt in Suzanne's mind. They were all there for Frank. Something horrible was happening to him.

After what must have seemed like a lifetime to Suzanne, Irene came back. There was another nurse and a doctor with her. "Mrs. Tomaso," the doctor began softly. "I'm so sorry." Suzanne stood up and started to scream. "No, no," she sobbed. "Don't tell me. I don't want to hear this! I won't listen to what you have to tell me! Don't do it! Please don't do it!" And with that Suzanne started to vomit into the artificial potted

53

plant standing in the corner of the room. By now all three kids were screaming alor
with her.

Irene had been an emergency room nurse for over ten years. She had seen a l
of tragedy and many people die. She had been present when hundreds of famili
learned that they had lost someone they loved very much. And of course, every sing
time that happened, Irene had been affected. But never like this. Irene did
understand it. Maybe it because Suzanne was her age and Frank had been as old as h
own husband. And Irene also had three kids who were just like the Tomaso kids
Maybe that was why.

That night Irene couldn't sleep at all. She kept looking at her husband and gettir
up to check on her kids. And when she saw the obituary in the newspaper, she felt eve
worse. Frank had become even more of a real person to her.

Irene never stopped thinking about what happened. Suzanne and Frank ar
those kids were on her mind every single day. She dreamed about them, and she relive
the scene in the emergency room over and over again. She was certain that Suzann
had lost her mind or killed herself or something. When Thanksgiving came and the
Christmas time, all Irene could think of was that family. She pictured them sitting an
crying all day. It got so bad that she considered getting some professional help f
herself. The Tomaso family never left Irene's mind.

And then winter turned to spring. Easter came and went, and although Irene wa
better, she still worried and wondered. Was that family alright, or had they fallen apar
Then, one lovely day in early May, Irene went to a big flea market in the parking lot of
big arena. It was one of those flea markets with hundreds of vendors and rows an
rows of tables.

Turning the corner at the end of one of the booths, suddenly Irene saw them.
was the Tomaso family, Suzanne and the three kids. They were with another youn
woman and two other children, and all five kids were running up and down the aisle
laughing and playing. Suzanne and her friend were also laughing. Suzanne carried
big tote bag, stuffed with items she had bought. She had gotten a perm and looke
terrific. They were all obviously having a great time.

Irene shrank back, not knowing what to say. Suzanne looked right at her an
smiled. She kept on walking and talking to her friend, and obviously had no idea wh
Irene was. Irene just stood there. As she waited, she suddenly felt as if she had bee
relieved of a great burden. Sighing out loud, Irene almost skipped down the aisle. Sh
felt wonderful.

Life goes on.

The Big Glass Room

The building was very old, and had been built as a sanitarium for tuberculosis patients. In those days, T.B. patients were isolated from the rest of the world and kept or months or even years, treated with large doses of fresh air and sunshine. That's what illed the T.B. bugs, they believed.

So all the sanitariums had sundecks where the patients were brought in the ummertime, and solariums where they spent the winter days. The solariums were ituated at the ends of the long corridors, and were big round rooms with tremendous lass windows instead of walls. That's where the healing sunshine came through, and om the outside of the buildings it looked as if there were rows of bubbles on the end of ach of the floors. In effect, these rooms were round glass balls.

Now, many years later, the building had been renovated and was used as a large cute care city hospital. And this particular solarium had become the twenty-two bed ecovery room. The solarium, like all the others, was drafty and cold in the winter, ince the frigid wind came right in between the panes of glass. In the summer, it was tifling since the bright hot sunshine created a greenhouse effect, much like what appens in a closed automobile on a hot sunny day. But, like all the old public hospitals n big cities, this one continued to be a busy facility, one which usually ran at full apacity.

One pleasant late spring evening, Becky, Laura, and Christie were on duty in that ecovery room. Even though the unit was full, it really wasn't too bad a shift. The room aced the west, and so, even at seven o'clock the fading daylight still shone in brightly hrough the glass walls.

Back then, there were no I.V. bags. Big glass bottles, just like those used today or hyperalimentation, held all solutions. There also was no such things as piggy backs or antibiotics, and so all the medications were mixed together in those same glass oottles. Penicillin, vitamins, potassium -- you name it, and they were added. iverything was considered to be compatible with everything else, and the routine was o mix these bottles for the next couple of shifts and then line them up on the metal tands which stood at the foot of each bed. So each bed had an array of different olored bottles arranged in strategic order.

Besides the I.V. bottles, nasogastric tubes drained into glass bottles and chest ubes drained their bright blood into underwater drainage setups made of three bottles

55

which were connected by rubber tubing. So the green bile, the red blood and the yello
multivitamins made quite a colorful arrangement in their glass bottles which we
everywhere in the big glass room. And with the reflection from the sun, it really w
quite pretty.

Laura and Becky were taking vital signs and Christie was sitting at the des
charting. Laura was leaning over the patient right next to Mr. Calabro when
suddenly sat up straight and then bolted from his stretcher. In an instant, he ripped o
his I.V. and his nasogastric tube and tore off his gown. Stark naked, Mr. Calabro bega
running in circles along the stretcher beds which lined the round room. His eyes we
glazed and he obviously had no idea where he was or what he was doing.

Suddenly, Mr. Calabro grabbed one of those yellow I.V. bottles. He lifted it u
and held it in front of his face, seemingly transfixed by the light shining through th
colored fluid. Then he looked up toward the big glass window at the head of th
patient's stretcher, and raised his arm like a pitcher taking his wind-up. As the nurse
stood frozen, Mr. Calabro swung his arm and let the bottle go. The weight of the heav
bottle sent it crashing into and right through the pane, splintering glass everywhere
Without any hesitation, he picked up the next bottle and did the same. And then he di
it again. And again. Through one window. And the next one. And the next one.

By the time the nurses could recover enough to move, Mr. Calabro had heave
the seventh bottle through the fourth window. There were still plenty of bottles and lo
of windows left. Most of the patients in that room were still fast asleep, so not many c
them even responded. But the nurses did. They did what probably a lot nurses woul
do in that situation. They ran.

Becky, Laura, and Christie turned and flew right out of that recovery roon
leaving all their patients alone with the naked maniac. Screaming for help, they ra
down the hall, with the sounds of breaking glass echoing up and down the corridor i
the background. Before anything else could happen, a young man appeared at the doc
of the recovery room. He was from the laundry department, and had just rolled the bi
linen cart out of the elevator and onto the floor.

Without any hesitation at all, the young man walked into the recovery room an
over to the crazed patient, who at that exact moment, was bending down to lift up
bloody drainage bottle which was attached to the chest of a fresh thoracotomy patient.
"Hi, pal," the young man said matter of factly to Mr. Calabro. "How about you and m
going out for a beer?" Mr. Calabro turned and looked at the young man. Releasing hi
hold on the big red bottle, he nodded and said, "That sounds good to me. Let's go."

The two men left the recovery room together. Mr. Calabro obviously had n
idea where he was, what he was doing, or that he was as naked as the day he was born
They walked down the hall, and as they arrived at the next nurses' station, Mr. Calabro

as grabbed from behind by two security guards who had just arrived on the floor. He as tied to a stretcher and then sedated. The hero laundry man simply said, "So long," d left the floor.

When he finally woke up, Mr. Calabro had absolutely no memory of what he had ne. The educated guess as to what had happened was that he had reacted to the avy dose of barbiturates he had received as premedication for his surgery.

All the patients had to be transferred from the glass recovery room until repairs to ose windows were made. It was quite a project. As for the three nurses, they were iticized for running out of the room instead of staying to protect their patients. But as any said, nobody knows how people react until they are in that same situation.

The round room continued to be used as a recovery room for the next two years til the new twenty story building was built. But to this day, those three nurses have t forgotten the sound of those big glass bottles crashing through those big glass indows of the big glass room. And they wonder what they would do if something like at ever happens again.

Mouthwash

The lady was in kidney failure. Her blood values were terrible and she was making just a little bit of urine. And she felt sick. Very sick.

They all knew Mrs. Palmer had a prolapsed uterus. That was nothing new. She ad used a pessary for years, as a lot of old ladies did. Inserted high up into the vagina, literally kept her uterus up where it belonged. But she had done without the pessary uring these past few years that she had been living in the nursing home. She really idn't care if everything slipped down, she said. It didn't matter.

They began the usual testing, the kind they always do when someone's kidney's egin to fail. The very first test, the I.V.P., showed that there was some kind of a echanical obstruction to both ureters. They were being pinched off, causing reflux of rine back up to the kidneys. The flow of urine needed to be opened up, one way or nother.

So they called a urologist. They were sure Mrs. Palmer was going to need to ave nephrostomies done in order to make a pathway for the urine to come out of the idneys. Preparing to examine the patient, Dr. Borland pulled back the covers. There n the draw sheet, right between her legs, was the lady's uterus. It had totally prolapsed nd, still attached of course, it had come completely out of her body.

Zenda was the nurse with Dr. Borland. She had seen a partially prolapsed uterus efore, but never one like this. At first Zenda thought she was looking at a decubitus or edsore the uterus had gotten from rubbing against the sheet, but then Zenda realized lat the circular thing in the center was the cervix. Very creepy.

Well, Dr. Borland had his diagnosis. He knew what was causing Mrs. Palmer's idney failure. The uterus had been pulling down so hard that it had taken the ureters vith it, bending them at such an angle that urine could no longer come through. It was bvious. Mrs. Palmer didn't need a urologist. She needed a gynecologist.

So a GYN consult was called. By this time it was eight o'clock at night. Dr.)'Leary came in to see the patient. Mrs. Palmer, oblivious to the fact that her uterus ras lying peacefully in bed with her, was now semi-conscious from the high levels of xins circulating in her bloodstream. As soon as he saw what had happened, Dr.)'Leary knew that in order to open up her kidneys, the uterus needed to be pushed back a and up. And an old fashioned pessary would do just fine.

58

But there it was, late in the evening. Where, oh where, was the doctor going get a pessary? Pessaries weren't exactly kept on supply carts, you know. So D O'Leary thought for a few seconds and then reached toward Mrs. Palmer's bedsic table. He picked up the mouthwash bottle, which was one of those small bottles fille with Cepacol. "This will do just fine," he said.

With a gloved hand, Dr. O'Leary picked up the pink uterus and pushed it slow but firmly back up towards where it belonged. As Zenda watched in disbelief, he the took that Cepacol mouthwash bottle and inserted it as far up Mrs. Palmer's vagina as would go. "Dr. O'Leary," mumbled Zenda, "Don't you want to dump out tl mouthwash first?" The gynecologist told her that the weight of the liquid made it stronger pessary, and so it was better to keep it full. When he let go, everything staye in place. Unbelievable.

He then suggested to Zenda that she might want to put a sanitary pad with a be on Mrs. Palmer, so in case everything should start to slip again, the bottle would k braced against the pad and it wouldn't come all the way out. Very clever, Zenc thought.

After Dr. O'Leary had left, the nurses started to think about what would happen the cap of the bottle got loose and the mouthwash spilled out inside of Mrs. Palmer The most that could happen, they laughed, is that Mrs. Palmer would get a Cepaco douche. And that shouldn't be a problem.

Well, this happened to be a Friday night, so no plans were made for Mr Palmer's future care. The only thing done was to order some more blood chemistries t be drawn in the morning. And lo and behold, they were much improved. With tl weight of that uterus off her urinary structures, Mrs. Palmer once again began to mak urine. By Sunday morning she was pretty much awake but had no idea that she had bottle filled with yellow mouthwash up inside of her. And the nurses chose not to te her.

That evening, as Zenda was feeding Mrs. Palmer her dinner, the lady began t cough and choke. Zenda had a feeling about what was going to happen, and when Mr Palmer called out, Zenda just knew she was right. She pulled back the sheets and then it was. Or rather, there *they* were. The mouthwash bottle and the uterus, lying togethe peacefully on the sheet.

So off Zenda went to the phone to call Dr. O'Leary, who was sorry he was o call this particular weekend. "Look, Zenda," he sighed. "You saw what I did. It wasr any big deal. Can you do it for me?" Zenda laughed. "No way," she said. I do a lot c things I shouldn't, but I draw the line at replacing organs." Dr. O'Leary laughed with he and asked her to call the house doctor.

59

By this time, Zenda was in a laughing fit. She called the house doctor. House doctors are usually called for a lot of reasons. They draw blood that the lab can't get. They evaluate patients who are having trouble breathing. They give certain medications. But it is very doubtful that many house doctors have ever been asked to place a prolapsed uterus and follow it up there with a loaded mouthwash bottle.

So the house doctor answered Zenda's request by telling her she was out of her mind and he was not going to do anything as unorthodox and crazy as that, even if he thought she was telling him the truth, which he didn't.

Well, anyway, Dr. O'Leary came back to the hospital late that Sunday night to do the mouthwash trick again. And, no the nurses didn't give him the same slimy bottle; they threw it in the garbage and gave him a brand new one. Filled, of course, with Cepacol. Later on that week, Mrs. Palmer was stable enough to undergo a hysterectomy, and yes, she went off to the operating room with the bottle still in place. There was a bit of laughter in the O.R. that day.

Mrs. Palmer did very well and was no longer in kidney failure. She was sent back to her nursing home, probably none the wiser about the close relationship she had developed with Cepacol mouthwash.

The Fever

She hadn't been to Atlantic City for about two months, and now today was finally the day. Carrie always started to get excited a little while before they left home. She got, in fact, what she called "the fever."

Every so often she read about those people who won the Megabucks or the Quartermania jackpot, and she always believed that if they could do it, so could she. Carrie only played the quarter machines, since being the great loser that she usually was, her money disappeared much too fast. Once in a while, in fact, she even played the nickel machines. That was when her trusty quarters were simply disappearing too fast.

Well, anyway, today was the day, and Carrie had "the fever." The feeling got stronger as they drove along the Atlantic City Expressway and she was able to see the skyline of all the casino hotels in the distance. They were calling to her.

Carrie had heartburn. She had heartburn on and off for many years and had been treating herself for it from day one. It got better and worse and then better again. Sometimes the heartburn woke her up as many as six or seven times a night, and so she kept a supply of medications right on her nightstand. Rolaids, Tums, Mylanta, Maalox, and her trusty favorite, Pepto Bismol, decorated her room. She chugged the Pepto right from the bottle. Sometimes, when it got bad, she even had to sleep propped straight up. So she was a pro at this.

Like a lot of nurses, Carrie never went to a doctor. What for? So that they could send her for a G.I. series and tell her that she had reflux esophagitis? That she should eat small bland feedings, not eat late at night, cut down on the caffeine (yeah, right!) and all the other stuff they tell people? She knew all of that. Anyway, she'd lived with this for fifteen years or so and she was very much alive. She knew how to treat herself, and now that Tagamet and Pepcid were sold over the counter, she would do even better.

Well, like most people with this aggravating condition, Carrie's stomach acid really started to churn when she was excited. And going to Atlantic City to take a couple of million or so away from Donald Trump certainly made her excited. "The fever" sure did increase her stomach acid production. She expected it. But Carrie had her usual bag full of antacids in the car with her; she never left home without her goody bag. So it wasn't a problem.

61

It was a little before noon when Carrie's husband suggested stopping for lunch They were only a few minutes from the casinos, but they were getting hungry. That wa a really good idea, Carrie thought. That way she wouldn't waste any of her preciou gambling time by having to stop and eat. They pulled into a Wendy's and backed int one of the few empty spaces. It was crowded inside but Wendy's lines always move fast. She loved Wendy's food and the service was good.

Lots of people were eating in their cars, Carrie saw. She always liked to g inside though. That way they could jump up to get extra ketchup and napkins and stuf like that. Carrie's husband got out of the car and started towards the entrance door. Waving at him to go ahead, Carrie decided to prepare her stomach for her hamburge and fries. Opening her bag, she dug around until she touched the familiar Pepto Bismo bottle. She should have stock in the stuff, she figured. She sure drank enough of it.

Opening the bottle, Carrie lifted the bottle to her lips. Naturally, it was the larg economy size. Just as she began to take a gigantic gulp, she caught a glimpse of th woman in the next car. The lady was looking at her with a funny expression on he face. Suddenly Carrie had a vision of a movie crew shooting a commercial for Wendy' and catching her chugging Pepto Bismol straight from the bottle. What horribl publicity that would be; obviously everyone would think she was drinking the stuf because of the food she had eaten. The lady in the next car probably did.

The thought of the Wendy's commercial made Carrie start to laugh. However since swallowing and laughing at the exact same second don't work too well, Carri proceeded to aspirate the Pepto Bismol. The lady in the next car, who was still starin at Carrie, was treated to a vision of this maniac with the pink bottle coughing an choking and gagging and then proceeding to spurt the pink liquid out from her nose.

The lady jumped out of the car, signaling wildly at a man just exiting from a ca parked farther down the row. They both began to beat at Carrie's car door, which sh had locked when all of this started. Sure that Carrie was most likely dying or havin some sort of seizure, the man ran back to his car and started honking madly for help. By this time Carrie once again had a decent air exchange. Pink tinged snot wa dripping from her nose and her face was streaked with tears, but she was breathing. She couldn't talk yet without coughing and her blue jacket was covered with pink blotches, but she was alive and frantically trying to motion those people to get awa from her. "I'm fine," she managed to squeak. "I'm a nurse." Like that would make a difference, Carrie moaned to herself. She probably had set the profession back a hundred years by this stunt.

A crowd had formed around the car by this time and Carrie just prayed that some good samaritan had not dialed 911 on his cellular phone. She could just imagine the police and paramedics arriving to save her. Oh, she would just die of embarrassment!

She wanted to start up the car and zoom out of the parking lot but her husband was inside on the line. She could see him through the plate glass window, standing there waiting for her.

After what seemed like an eternity, the people started to walk away from the car inside which Carrie remained barricaded. She had no tissues or napkins and was forced to mop up her dripping nose and eyes with the vomit covered jacket. Oh, God, she was so disgusting looking! Finally, her husband stuck his head out the door to see what had happened to Carrie. Unable to call to him without hacking and choking, she motioned wildly for him to come to the car. When he opened the door, he was treated to the sight and smell of his dripping, blotchy, pathetic wife who grabbed his arm and croaked, "Drive! Go! I'll explain later!"

Ten minutes later they pulled into the parking lot of a McDonalds. Carrie's stinky jacket had been rolled into a ball and stuffed into the trunk. No longer coughing, she was ready to eat. She knew they would never be able to return to that Wendy's again, even though that was where they always stopped on the way to Atlantic City. Her picture would most likely be posted in the crazy person's section or something. Oh, well, now it was time to stuff herself so that she would be full of energy when she won her millions. Popping a spearmint flavored Rolaid into her mouth, they got out of the car. Boy, those fries smelled good! She'd have a big lunch then have some mylanta for dessert.

"The fever" was back.

Maggots

The lady was comatose. For years she had fought a battle with cancer which had begun in the roof of her mouth and had spread up and through her sinuses. Surgery and radiation had not stopped the growth of the virulent tumor, and now she had suffered a major stroke.

Mrs. Jenkins was admitted to the intensive care unit. She was on a respirator and was doing very little in the way of breathing on her own. The lady had lots of mucus coming out of her nose and mouth, as well as from her endotracheal tube. The secretions were thick and foul smelling, and the doctors believed that the cancer was causing infection in her sinuses.

Well, it was six o'clock in the morning, the day after Mrs. Jenkins' admission. As was the routine in that unit, the night nurses did some of the baths and morning care. So Debbie went into the room and filled the bath basin. Before beginning the bath, she prepared to suction Mrs. Jenkins. The room was dim, the light coming from the hall. Debbie saw what she thought was a shadow on Mrs. Jenkins' face, across her upper lip. Debbie switched on the light just in time to see a small white worm sticking out of Mrs. Jenkins' left nostril. As soon as the light hit it, the worm wiggled quickly back up her nose.

At first Debbie couldn't believe what she was seeing. She stood there frozen and then let out a little moan. Then she turned around and left the room. She didn't scream or yell or anything like that, although when she thought about it later she couldn't understand why she hadn't done so. Walking quickly out to the nurses' station, she grabbed her friend Lauren by the hand and pulled her into the medication room. A new patient had just been admitted and his whole family was right there in the middle of the unit, so she had to try to be calm.

"Lauren," whispered Debbie hoarsely. "I saw a worm crawl up Mrs. Jenkins' nose! I'm not crazy! I really did! And I'm telling you right now, Lauren," Debbie added, "I am never ever going back in that room again!"

Lauren just looked at Debbie. "Do you mean like a maggot? Is that what you're saying?" she asked. Debbie started to get a little wild. "How do I know what it was?" she asked, her voice becoming shrill. "Do you think I am some kind of a worm expert or something? It was a worm, a gross, disgusting, white worm and I saw it crawl up that lady's nose! Oh, my God. Oh, my God!"

Well, none of the nurses on the night shift went back into the room. The watched Mrs. Jenkin's cardiac rhythm and her vital signs on the monitor, but they a knew that even if she had a cardiac arrest or something, they was no way that they wer going to get close to her. It was lucky she stayed stable.

So the day shift arrived and they told the worm story. Most of the staff reacte just as Debbie and her pals did, but Jane, for some unknown reason, volunteered to tak care of Mrs. Jenkins. She said she felt like having a "different" sort of day.

She got it.

Jane saw a worm the first time she approached the bed. It was hanging out o her patient's nose. Instead of screaming, Jane laughed out loud, calling, "Look, look! It's the worm!" But little did Jane know that *the* worm really was *many* worms. Because once that worm ventured out in the light, he brought with him his entire family It was so gross, they all said. Just imagine going in to take care of a critically ill patien on a ventilator and finding a pile of white wiggly worms crawling all over her face.

Gag.

So an ear, nose, and throat specialist was called in and it didn't take long to fin an explanation. It seems the cancer in the maxillary sinuses had become necrotic. Necrotic tissue is dead tissue, and maggots come from dead tissue. The only problem was that the rest of Mrs. Jenkins' body was still alive. The E.N.T. doctor very calmly looked up her nose, and by the light of his trusty headlamp and with the help of a long forceps, extracted five or six wiggly white maggots. He placed them in a specimen cup and told Jane to send them to the lab. Jane, by this time, had stopped laughing.

Mrs. Jenkins lived only one more day. It would be very nice to say her nursing care remained constant and complete, but that would be a big fat lie. Unfortunately, the nurses who were assigned to take care of her gave just the absolute minimum and stayed out of her room as much as possible. And everyone understood why.

Three days later, somebody wondered if the undertaker should have been told that a family of worms could come out of her nose or mouth at any time. And what it her family was viewing her body at the wake and the worms decided to take a little walk? But since undertakers deal with dead bodies all the times, they decided that it wasn't necessary. The embalming fluid would kill worms, wouldn't it? And if it didn't, shouldn't the morticians should know how to handle maggots?

And if they didn't, there was nothing anyone could do about it now, anyway.

Failure

It was a little after eleven at night, and a group of them were leaving the hospital. Carolyn hadn't felt very well that day; she had been conscious of a vague headache along with some kind of pressure in the back of her neck. It was different than anything she had experienced before.

Carolyn was young and newly married. She worked the evening shift, but was waiting for a position on days to open up. After all, she wanted to be home at night with her new husband. They missed each other.

So the nurses continued out to the parking lot and spread out as they reached their cars. Suddenly, without making a sound, Carolyn collapsed on the ground. There was no warning, no nothing. One second she was waving goodbye, and the next she was not there any more. She was dead.

One of the nurses ran back, screaming, towards the hospital in an effort to get help. The other two began to do C.P.R., crying out loud as they were working. There was no breathing and no pulse. Nothing. No sign of life.

After what seemed like an eternity, a crowd of people came running out to the parking lot. There were E.M.T's, paramedics, nurses, and two resident physicians. They jumped on Carolyn and intubated her right there on the ground. They shocked her and gave her drugs and put in I.V. lines on the cold hard concrete floor, and then they put her in the ambulance that had come out to the lot. Carolyn was brought into the emergency department and put in a trauma room. The code continued for more than an hour. Everybody was there and everything was tried.

Carolyn never regained any kind of a heart rhythm. She never took a breath. She never moved or flinched or showed any kind of reflex. She had, for all purposes, died out there on the parking lot floor just as she was saying goodbye to her friends. The autopsy showed a massive intra-cerebral bleed caused by the rupture of a huge aneurysm. She didn't have a chance.

Being in the right place at the right time meant nothing. She had all the skills and all the equipment at hand, and nothing could help her. Carolyn's funeral service was standing room only. Besides all the people who knew her and loved her, those who tried to save her were there too. It's hard to explain the mixed feelings. Some people were still angry, saying that maybe they could have done something else or something more. But deep down, they must have known that there had been nothing left to do.

Carolyn will not be forgotten in that hospital. She stands for a wish that could not come true, no matter how hard people tried. Sometimes when a particularly sad c tragic event takes place, people look at each other and simply say, "Remembe Carolyn." And they think of just how fragile a life can be.

The Big Red Lollypop

Even with the tube feedings and the hyperalimentation, the kid was still starving. A young man in his twenties, Brian had been severely injured in an auto accident. The extent of the damage to his brain profoundly affected his ability to speak and swallow.

His gag and cough reflexes were very weak, and Brian still had a tracheostomy. He needed to be suctioned because he was unable to cough effectively enough to clear his airway. The few times Brian was given swallowing trials, he aspirated. Everyone hoped that all this would improve, but it was going to take a great deal of time.

Brian's room was always filled with visitors. He was a very popular person and, even after his accident, his friends never let him down. Sometimes the guys came straight from work, and they ate their dinners in Brian's room. Family members also snacked while they spent time with Brian. Coffee and buns and doughnuts were standard, and it was obvious that the smell of food made Brian even more hungry. Finally, everyone decided not to eat in front of Brian; it frustrated him that he wasn't able to swallow anything.

One day, one of Brian's nurses decided that even though he was unable to swallow food, he should still be allowed to taste it. So she had an idea. Janet would get him something that he could suck on, something that would still permit him to experience flavor. She couldn't give him something that he would be able to chew, because if he tried to do so he could choke. So Janet went down to the gift shop and bought a big red lollypop. She picked it not only for its color and flavor, but also for its size. There was no way that Brian could chew that great big thing, so it would be safe as well as delicious and satisfying.

Janet brought the big lollypop up to the floor and showed it to Brian. "Look what I got for you, Brian," Janet announced excitedly. "It's cherry flavored and I'll bet it's delicious." She peeled off the colored wrapper and held the lollypop in front of Brian's face. "Here you go, Brian," Janet said. "Lick it." Brian broke out in a big smile. It was obvious that he couldn't wait to taste that big red lollypop. He took a few small licks, savoring the flavor. It had been a long time since he had eaten anything at all, and this obviously tasted great. Suddenly, Brian opened his mouth wide, and a split second later he chomped down on that gigantic red lollypop and broke half of it off. Before Janet had a chance to react, Brian took a big gulp and swallowed. The red lollypop disappeared.

Suddenly, Brian began to cough. But since his cough reflex was so weak, Brian did nothing more than make short ineffective attempts at clearing his airway. At first Janet thought that Brian had swallowed that big piece of lollypop, and simply had some minor irritation from sensing something in the back of his throat. After all, it had been quite some time since he had eaten anything. Not wanting to believe what she knew had really happened, Janet told herself that maybe it was the unfamiliar feeling which was making him cough like that. But within seconds it became obvious that something was very wrong. Brian's color was changing and he couldn't stop those coughs, which were now becoming more and more like short little gasps.

Janet looked into Brian's open mouth. There was nothing there. No trace of the big red lollypop. At this point, Janet got an icy feeling in the pit of her stomach. It was now very clear what had happened. That lollypop had gone down, all right. It had gone directly down into Brian's trachea. Janet grabbed for the wall suction. She stuck the plastic catheter in Brian's mouth, pushing it down Brian's throat. Janet had no idea what she was doing, since it was quite obvious that the soft little number fourteen tube was not going to vacuum up a gigantic chunk of candy. All the catheter did was stimulate Brian's weak gag reflex. And through all of this, he continued with his poor attempt to cough. And nothing, of course, came up.

As luck would have it, a pulmonologist was sitting out in the nurses' station writing in a chart. He was not involved in Brian's case, but heard Janet's calls for help. Dr. Hillman jumped up and immediately ran into the room. Calling for a laryngoscope, he opened Brian's mouth and retracted his tongue. He saw nothing.

At this point, Janet lost it. She ran out of the room, crying out loud that she had killed her patient. The other nurses went in to help Dr. Hillman. Janet left the unit and escaped into the nurses' locker room, where she sat huddled in the corner, her back against the wall. Janet stayed there for what seemed like an eternity, listening to the STAT pages for respiratory therapy, any ear, nose, throat physicians, and finally for any thoracic surgeon. By this time, Janet was hysterical. She was sure Brian was dead or dying and she knew it was all her fault.

Finally, a lifetime later, one of the nurses came in to get Janet. "He's O.K.," she said, reaching out towards the sobbing nurse. "Dr. Hillman got it out. And Brian is all right." Very slowly, Janet walked out of the locker room and back into the unit. Dr. Hillman was there, all covered with perspiration. He looked at Janet and smiled. "I saw it there," he said quietly. "It was right below the vocal chords. I saw it. It was big and bright red and shiny and was bobbing up and down with each breath. I just couldn't get it. I never thought I'd get it in time, but finally I was able to grab it with the McGill Forceps. I got it. I got it. I finally got it."

Janet looked at the desk. There was a specimen jar on the counter, the kind that holds urine and mucus and other stuff that gets sent to the lab. And there in the jar was the big red lollypop. There was nothing that Janet could say to Dr. Hillman. She just looked at him and shook her head. He put his arms around her and hugged her tightly. As horrible as it had been for everyone, Dr. Hillman knew it had been worse for Janet. He knew, as she did, that if Brian had died, Janet could never have practiced nursing again. As much of an accident as it was, that would have been the end.

"If you hadn't been here - - - " Janet started to say. Dr. Hillman interrupted her. "But I was," he said kindly. "And it's over." Janet walked slowly into Brian's room. His color was pink and he was breathing easily. He looked at Janet and smiled. Janet touched his cheek and then bent down and kissed it. She turned and left his room to pull herself together.

As far as Janet was concerned, from that day on Dr. Hillman was Janet's guardian angel. The report from the pathology lab came back and very simply stated, "foreign body removed from trachea." And it was quite a while before Janet could bring herself to talk about the day her patient almost choked to death on the red lollypop that she had bought for him, and very much longer before she could write about it.

Tetanus

Nobody ever sees tetanus anymore, at least that's what they thought. But this man, a fifty year old who had been in excellent health, now was dying of the disease.

Mr. Tinton had sliced his finger on some kind of a garden tool, and he had developed tetanus. It had taken a while to diagnose him because the systemic symptoms could have been anything. But that piece of equipment had been old and coated with dried soil, and that's where they guessed the bacteria had come from. Mr. Tinton, like too many adults, hadn't received a tetanus shot in over twenty-five years.

The disease had progressed to the point that Mr. Tinton was on a ventilator. To nobody's surprise, the tetanus antitoxin hadn't helped. Mr. Tinton was in the later stages of the illness. The doctors had amputated his finger, but the toxin had already spread throughout the nervous system. Everyone knew he was going to die and the goal now was to keep Mr. Tinton comfortable and free of the painful spasms and tonic contractions that typified a tetanus infection. The patient was in the I.C.U., but it was an old unit, one with beds divided by curtains rather than individual rooms. There was, however, one private cubicle in the back of the unit and that was Mr. Tinton's. Blankets had been draped across the glass to keep the area as dark as possible, and there were signs all over the place urging silence. Any noise or movements were known to institute spasms. In fact, the simple act of someone brushing against the bed could set off a major event.

Mr. Tinton received regular doses of valium and pain medication but he slept only sporadically, and it was obvious when the rigid spasms set in. Patients with tetanus have an overactive sympathetic nervous system, and so everything speeds up. The goal in patients like these is to slow things down.

On this particular evening, Pat was taking care of Mr. Tinton. His physical care was kept to an absolute minimum, since even the slightest touch stimulated him. The nurses whispered to him when they came near to let them know they were at his bedside. Nobody wanted to startle him. So Pat was standing by Mr. Tinton's bed, getting ready to change his almost empty I.V. bottle. The lights were off, and it was difficult to see. Pat took the old bottle down and pulled the tubing from the hole. She took the new bottle and pushed the spike back in, and then reached up to hang it back on the pole. Somehow, the spike hadn't been secured in the opening, and in a split second the full and heavy glass bottle came crashing down onto the floor.

71

Instinctively, Pat jumped backwards. She knew the bottle was likely to splinter and shower her and everything else with the sharp shreds of glass which were coated with the fifty percent glucose based hyperalimentation solution. She was right. The bottle seemed to explode and disintegrate into a million slivers of wet and sticky glass particles. But when Pat moved to get out of the way, her backside slammed into Mr. Tinton's overbed table, on which a ton of equipment had been piled, as well as the empty I.V. bottle which Pat had just taken down. The table, on its rollers, slid backwards and then banged into the chair by the bed. Everything hit the floor. The noise was deafening.

Mr. Tinton's body arched backward in the classic pose of opisthotonos. Being on the ventilator, he couldn't make a sound, but even in the dark Pat could see the agony in his eyes. Pat grabbed his arm, most likely making things even worse. "Oh, God, Mr. Tinton," cried Pat. "I'm so sorry. I'm so sorry!"

By this time everyone had run back to the doorway of the cubicle. Someone turned the big overhead light on to see what had happened. There was glass and yellow liquid and supplies everywhere. And there was Pat, holding helplessly to the end of Mr. Tinton's I.V. tubing so that it wouldn't become contaminated. It was some awful scene.

Well, it took a long time to settle things down. They had to move Mr. Tinton out of that room so that the tremendous chaos could be cleaned up. Any nurse who has ever come in contact with dripping intravenous hyperalimentation knows exactly what a sticky mess it causes, and this particular mess was packed with broken glass. There was no way that anyone could continue to care for Mr. Tinton in that cubicle; the way things were it was not even possible to walk around in the room.

Mr. Tinton had to be brought into the big unit. They laid a bath towel across his eyes to try to keep the light out, even though the brightness was only a very small part of the stimuli of that big intensive care unit. It took quite a while and a lot of medication until those horrible tonic spasms dissipated. And it took even longer for Pat to forgive herself for what had happened.

The day after the event, Mr. Tinton died.

Doctor Kevin's Birthday

Dr. Kevin was the nurses' favorite resident. He was as nice as he was smart, and he was everyone's friend. When Dr. Kevin was working, he kept everyone laughing. Even the worst days turned out good if he was in the hospital. He had the greatest sense of humor and could see a joke in everything. Dr. Kevin was a stress buster and a nut.

At the end of his medical residency, Dr. Kevin was accepted at another hospital to start a fellowship in cardiology. He told the nurses that he'd be back as a staff cardiologist, and they knew he would.

True to his word, Dr. Kevin came back. And as everyone guessed, he was terrific. He was the same old Dr. Kevin, funny and crazy as ever. And he helped out all the other doctors by taking extra call and just covering when they needed a few hours off for something important.

Well, Dr. Kevin's thirtieth birthday was coming up and he really wanted the day off. But for a variety of reasons, he found himself on call for the emergency room, and for the same reasons he just couldn't get anyone to cover for him. Maybe, since his birthday fell on a Saturday, he thought to himself, he would be lucky and have some free hours. After all, Saturdays were usually easier than weekdays. Then he could celebrate his birthday after all. Think positive, he told himself.

Yeah, right.

It first hit the fan on Friday night. He was called in on consult to see a patient who had just had abdominal surgery. Both the man's legs had turned blue from the waist down. So into the Recovery Room went Dr. Kevin. The man was in shock. He was in kidney failure. He was in metabolic acidosis. He had multiple cardiac arrhythmias. He was septic. He had developed clotting disorders and was bleeding to death. The cuff on his endotracheal tube was leaking and he needed to be reintubated. He needed a pulmonary artery catheter. And so on. And as soon as Dr. Kevin dealt with one crisis, the next one arose.

This patient was eight-six years old and had a gangrenous bowel. He was going to die, and that was certain. Dr. Kevin made seven trips out to the waiting room to try to get a "Do Not Resuscitate" order, but the family wouldn't hear of it. "He's strong, Doc," they told him. "Don't give up." So Dr. Kevin worked on and on into the night, until the patient finally coded and died at three o'clock in the morning. His birthday morning.

By the time Dr. Kevin got home and got into bed, it was after four. At seven o'clock, the phone rang. It was the emergency room and they had another disaster in progress. It seemed there was a fifty year old man who had come in during the night saying he had a "funny feeling in his chest." Well, he'd been worked up completely and they'd found nothing. Certainly nothing related to his heart, and so he was discharged home.

The man had gone to the bathroom while his wife went out to get the car. And while he was in the bathroom, his heart had stopped. He was clinically dead. But of course, people who become clinically dead in an emergency room certainly are not left that way, so the circus had begun. The emergency room doctor, when she called Dr. Kevin, told him that this man was going to need a bunch of procedures to keep him from dying. They needed a cardiologist STAT. And guess who was still on call?

Well, Dr. Kevin was always an impeccable dresser, and the day of his thirtieth birthday certainly was not going to be any exception. So Dr. Kevin put on his brand new Armani suit, which he had bought specifically to wear on his birthday, and raced to the emergency room just in time to find the staff working on the guy like crazy. The cardiogram showed that the man, who was now wild and fighting the respirator, was right in the middle of having a massive heart attack. He had almost no blood pressure and was on a bunch of intravenous drips.

The patient obviously needed to receive T.P.A., the famous "clot buster", and they had already brought him into the procedure room for the pulmonary artery catheter. But he was bleeding like crazy from his nose, since they had had a terrible time intubating him and had gouged up the back of his throat with the laryngoscope blade. Dr. Kevin weighed the pros and cons of giving T.P.A. to a bleeding patient, and decided that it needed to be given. So they hung the drug.

Then holding the introducer for the P.A. catheter in his hand, Dr. Kevin prayed out loud, "Oh, please, God, let me get this on one stick so I don't have to make lots of holes in his chest and kill him with the T.P.A." The introducer and the catheter went right in. This is a sign that things will be O.K. now, thought Dr. Kevin.

Sure. Dream on.

Well, now it was time to put in the temporary pacemaker wire, because the patient, although awake, was now in complete heart block. So picture this. Doctor Kevin, who never even had time to take off his suit jacket before all this started, was leaning over the poor patient. He was just about to start the pacer procedure, when the patient pointed to his belly. As Dr. Kevin began to ask if his stomach hurt, the patient turned his head directly towards him, and projectile vomited what seemed to be a gallon of undigested corn and chicken (mixed with a moderate amount of blood) right over Dr. Kevin and his brand new Armani suit.

Doctor Kevin, with a loud howl, jumped back from the bed just as the second wave of the undigested blood soaked dinner shot forth and landed squarely in the E.R. nurse's face and on top of her head. As she screamed out loud, Dr. Kevin kneeled down and began to pick the corn niblets out of his expensive Italian shoes.

So instead of going ahead with the pacemaker insertion, there was a short break while Doctor Kevin scrubbed madly at his suit with combines soaked in peroxide, and the nurse stuck her head under the running water in the sink, letting the clumps of chicken and corn run down and stuff up the drain. And of course the poor patient was helplessly watching the entire episode.

Well, before the pacemaker was finally inserted and the patient's cardiac rhythm stabilized, the patient had vomited up three bedpans with much of the same. Doctor Kevin wanted to ask the family if the patient had eaten dinner from a plate or simply fed out of a trough. But he controlled himself.

By the time this whole nightmare was over, it was noontime on the birthday Saturday, and Dr. Kevin had a whole bunch of patients waiting for him to see. He wound up changing into scrubs and stuffing his classy suit into a plastic garbage bag to take to the cleaners to see if they could save it. Dr. Kevin worked straight through until ten o'clock that night, and truly it was one of the worst two days he had ever had. He fell into bed and went to sleep the very minute he got home.

Happy birthday, Dr. Kevin.

By the way, the suit was saved but the patient died.

The Regis Diner

It was a dark and stormy night, as the stories say. The skies had opened up and it was teeming. But that didn't stop the group from doing their thing.

Just as they had been doing for years, they left the hospital together to go out to eat. Every night for as long as they could remember, the evening shift went out to the Regis Diner. The Regis had everything, from hamburgers to pizza to eggs. Open 24 hours a day, the Regis was a very popular spot for the hospital family. The late night crowd was made up mainly of young people. Nurses, interns and residents, respiratory therapists, and technologists and technicians. They all knew each other, and as permanent shift people tend to do, they had become very close. That's what happens in hospitals. Evening and night shift people have special bonds.

Well, as per their routines, the nurses took turns driving. It seemed silly for a bunch of cars to drive together and look for places to park. Since the Regis was barely a mile from the hospital, whoever was the driver drove his or her passengers back to the hospital and dropped them off in the parking lot after they ate. Then everyone went to their own cars and drove home. That's the way it worked, and this rainy summer night was no different.

The group of five nurses returned to the hospital shortly after one in the morning. The rain had let up, and although they could see lightning flashes in the distance, it was only drizzling. Waving goodbye, each of the girls ran to their cars. Now this was a very big hospital campus, made up of lots of buildings. And these building were spread out all over the grounds, with parking spaces almost everywhere. On this particular night, Gail's car was parked way in back of what was known as the powerhouse, a building which housed generators or machines or something like that. The grounds were pretty dark also, but for some reason, nobody ever was afraid to walk at night. Maybe it was because of the big high fence which surrounded the entire hospital complex. It usually felt safe.

So Gail ran behind the powerhouse and quickly got into her car. Boy, was this area deserted. And with the puddles blowing in the wind, it really looked scary. She was glad that she didn't have to fumble for her keys in the rain; the front door lock was broken and she never even thought about getting it fixed. What for? She was safe on the hospital grounds.

Yeah, right.

Gail threw her pocketbook on the seat next to her and unzipped her coat. She didn't like to drive with a coat on, since it made her feel cramped. And this was before the time of seatbelts. So Gail got herself comfortable in the front seat, and then fished around in her oversized pocketbook. She found the key and stuck it in the ignition. Gail started the car up and then went back into her bag for a stick of gum. It was a good couple of minutes before she was finally ready to leave. She put her foot on the brake and put the car into reverse. Then just before she began to back out of the parking space, she automatically glanced up at the rear view mirror. There was a man in her back seat.

Gail went nuts. In one split second she was out of the car. Her pocketbook left behind on the front seat, Gail ran screaming back toward the main hospital buildings. She ran like a crazy person, sliding and slipping in the mud and shrieking non stop. This was a huge county hospital with a police station based in the emergency room, and that's exactly where Gail was headed. By the time she reached the E.R., she looked like a mud wrestler. The thunderstorm was once again in its full glory, and God knows what people thought when they saw this slimy mud monster come barreling toward them, bellowing like a lunatic. And plenty of people were out there to witness this scene, since there was a group of E.R. people and cops standing out under the overhang watching the storm.

By the time Gail could speak and tell them that she was O.K. and had not been attacked or dragged through the weeds, quite a while passed. The policemen, although certain that the guy in the back seat was long gone, told Gail to get in their police car. Someone had enough brains to bring out a blanket for her to sit on so that the back seat of the patrol car would not become a swamp. They sped back to the powerhouse, and the cops jumped out and shone the light into Gail's car. There was the man, fast asleep in the back seat. The front door was still standing open and the pocketbook was there, untouched and just as Gail had left it. Obviously, Gail had been nothing more than an annoying pest to this poor man, who simply had wanted a place to sleep and to get out of the rain.

Anyway, the policemen took the guy back to the main police booth in the emergency room, and Gail followed in her car. They kept her there for quite a long time, filling out papers and having her answer a million questions. The sergeant even yelled at Gail like it was her fault for having a broken lock, telling her he was going to keep an eye out for her and give her some kind of a ticket if she didn't get it fixed. Gail had to call home and wake up her mother and tell her that she wouldn't be home until much later because she had found a man in the back seat of her car. Then she had to listen to her mother scream and yell and get her father all upset. But the worst part of everything was that the orthopedic resident who Gail had the hots for was right there in the emergency room and of course he saw Gail looking like the amazing mud man from hell. Absolutely mortifying.

Well, life went on. The group of evening shift people continued to go to the Regis Diner, and Gail went with them. She did, however, begin looking in through her car windows before she *unlocked* her door. And she began arriving at work a few minutes early so she wouldn't have to park behind the powerhouse any more. Today, a lifetime later, the Regis Diner is still standing and is still the hangout for the people of the evening shift. And every so often Gail thinks about these young doctors and nurses and wonders if they always lock their car doors.

Probably not.

Doctor God

They had just arrived at the candy machines when they heard the code for the cardiac arrest. It was about three o'clock in the morning. Jim and Marion, assigned to the medical I.C.U., knew it was meant for the new patient being transferred in from one of the general medical units. The man had had a stroke and had gotten progressively worse as the night went on.

At first the nurses stayed where they were, knowing that this would most likely be their one and only chance to get off the floor for any type of a break. Codes were routine in the critical care units, and the odds were that the two remaining nurses would have help from the I.C.U. next door. They'd manage O.K.

But after a few minutes, a different kind of call came over the public address system. The page came for any surgeon to report to the I.C.U. Jim and Marion took off for the stairs, knowing there was a problem.

On arrival in the unit, they found two residents and a group of nurses around one of the beds. It turned out that the patient had stopped breathing and nobody was able to get a tube down his trachea. They had been trying for the past twenty minutes, even before he was transferred into the I.C.U. And now, he was in big trouble.

Lots of times there are problems intubating people. And it seems that in Mr. Brown's case, a bunch of residents and paramedics had tried. And still nobody could get a tube down Mr. Brown's throat. He was being breathed, or rather attempted to be breathed, by an ambu bag attached to a mask which was clamped tightly over his nose and mouth. But very little air was entering Mr. Brown's lungs; it was obvious that there was some kind of obstruction in his trachea or vocal cords. And to top it off, all the attempts to insert a tube through that obstruction had caused swelling and inflammation which made everything much worse.

Well, it was quite obvious that the patient was not going to be intubated, and it was equally apparent that if an airway was not quickly established, he was going to die. Mr. Brown need to have an emergency tracheostomy.

Contrary to the episode of "M.A.S.H." in which Father Mulcahy performed a tracheostomy in the back seat of a jeep on a wounded soldier with the barrel of a ballpoint pen, there is a bit more involved than just making a hole. A tracheostomy should be done correctly and skillfully; you just don't stab someone in the neck. At least not in an intensive care unit.

79

So who was going to do the trach? At three o'clock in the morning, this hospital was not exactly crawling with surgeons ready and waiting to dash off to the intensive care unit. That left the residents, none of whom were exactly expert in doing emergency tracheotomies. And since a surgeon was needed, the first year surgical resident was put into the position of performing the trach. After all, he was probably the only physician who had ever been involved in the procedure before. And this great expertise probably consisted of holding the trach hooks a couple of times while the second and third year residents did the work under controlled operating room conditions. But any way you looked at it, he still had more experience than his first year colleagues in internal medicine. The senior surgical resident was paged, but it obviously was not possible to wait for him to wake up, put on his clothes, and get there instantaneously from three buildings away.

So the nurses opened the tracheostomy set and the young resident put on his gloves and got started. The poor guy's hands were shaking, but he knew he had to get an airway into this man and do it fast. The medical resident also put on a pair of gloves and tried to assist him, but he had absolutely no concept of what he was doing.

Jim and Marion were nurses who had been around for a long time, back when I.C.U. trachs were done at the bedside in order to spare the patient and staff the ordeal of traveling to the O.R. They had seen and assisted with more than a few bedside tracheostomies. And so it was obvious that they were the real experts on the scene. There is a saying that smart young doctors can learn a lot from smart nurses, and fortunately these guys knew it. The surgical resident tried to feel for the anatomical landmarks, but by this time Mr. Brown's pulse was dropping fast. "Hurry up," encouraged Marion. "He needs air, and fast."

The resident began the procedure and suddenly blood was everywhere. Jim and the medical resident were putting pressure on bleeding points as best as they could without getting their fingers in the way of that shaking scalpel. Marion had the suction catheter in the field, trying to suck as much blood out of the way as she could, so that the surgeon could see what he was doing. Once the blade actually penetrated the trachea, a small amount of air was sucked into it, since the patient was still desperately trying to breathe. The problem was that along with the air, the accumulating blood was also being drawn in and down into the lungs. The doctor was attempting to open the incision wider so that he could get the tracheostomy tube in place, when the senior surgical resident came racing into the unit.

"What the hell is going on here? What the hell do you think you're doing?" he yelled. "Leave him alone," Marion snapped back at him. "He's doing what he has to do to try to save this guy's life."

The senior resident positioned himself across from his junior colleague. He physically pushed the medical resident out of the way and started barking out orders. Get me gloves. Get me some more light. Give me some clamps." The nurses looked t each other and shook their heads. This doctor was known as a pompous ass with a god complex. Everyone hoped that when he finished his surgical residency, he would leave this hospital and not become a staff surgeon here. He would be absolutely impossible as an attending physician.

So Dr. God got the tube into the trachea after a lot of difficulty, yelling all the while that this was all the young resident's fault because he had made such a horrible incision. By the time the tube was tied in place, the room looked like a butcher shop. There was blood everywhere, including the curtains and the walls. The patient was now able to be breathed mechanically and was being adequately ventilated. The respirator was brought into the room and the patient hooked up to it. The senior resident never stopped complaining about the sloppy job that was done and the incompetence of the junior resident. When he finished and stepped away from the stretcher, he took a look at the patient for the first time and realized that Mr. Brown was comatose.

"Look what you did!" he yelled. "You created a goddamn living vegetable! You left him without oxygen for so long that you made him brain damaged. He's a goddamn cork, and it's all your fault! I'm not taking the rap for this one. You'll all answer for this!" For a minute nobody spoke. Then Jim began, carefully choosing his words. Listen, Doctor," he said softly. Mr. Brown had a big stroke a few hours earlier. He was like this before he was transferred into the I.C.U. He is not this way from lack of oxygen."

Dr. God glared at the group. "You damn well better be right," he said. Striding out of the unit, he left the entire team standing there in the middle of the mess. "I'm leaving," he announced to nobody in particular. "Do the paperwork." And then he was gone.

"Screw him," said the medical resident. "We did great. Let's clean up this mess and make some coffee."

And they did.

The Quiet Room

He was on the pulmonologist on call, and was just covering for the man's regular ⸱ctor. Dr. Julius took the phone call at home, just as he was about to sit down for his ⸱nner.

Mr. Toohey had just coded. A terminal lung cancer patient, his family had ⸱fused to listen to anyone, had denied that Mr. Toohey was going to die. "Just get him ⸱tter, Doc," they always said. "Just get him better."

So as sick as he was, and as hopeless as the situation had seemed, Mr. Toohey ⸱as treated as vigorously as could possibly be done. Although his personal physician ⸱ly believed that Mr. Toohey would not leave the hospital this time, he never told the ⸱mily that. He knew they didn't want to hear it and wouldn't listen.

Well, by the time Dr. Julius arrived on the floor, the code had been in full swing ⸱r over forty minutes. Dr. Julius checked the patient, made a quick review of what had ⸱en done, and then called the code. Mr. Toohey had obviously been dead since the ⸱ry beginning. Now the family had to be told.

So Dr. Julius walked out to the "quiet room", the area to which all families were ⸱ought when bad things happen and they need a place for private or confidential ⸱nversation. Tonight the quiet room was empty, except for the Toohey family. ⸱aving heard the code announced just as they were arriving to visit, they hadn't yet ⸱ached the unit. They knew that something was going on, that he had, in hospital talk, ⸱aken a turn for the worse." Dr. Julius opened the door to the quiet room. He came ⸱ce to face with two of the largest people he had ever seen.

The young man must have been in his middle twenties and probably weighed ⸱ound three hundred and fifty pounds. He easily stood six feet three or four. The ⸱oman, seated on the couch, was Mr. Toohey's wife. She seemed to be about the same ⸱ze. Now, Dr. Julius was a small man. He was no more than five feet six and weighed ⸱aybe a hundred forty pounds.

Dr. Julius closed the door behind him. He sat down on the couch next to Mrs. ⸱oohey, and motioned for the son to do the same. The young man, hesitating for just a ⸱oment, did so. "I'm so very sorry," began Dr. Julius. "Mr. Toohey has passed away. ⸱e all tried very hard but he just didn't make it."

A look of disbelief passed over the son's face, and was quickly replaced by one ⸱f horror and then rage. Rising slowly from his seat, the young man appeared to be growing larger right there on the spot. And then, as if in slow motion, he turned and leaned down over Dr. Julius. Grasping him by the lapels on his sports jacket, he pulled the doctor to his feet and then lifted him straight up into the air. He slammed Dr. Julius up against the corner of the wall and said very softly, "You killed my father and now I'm going to kill you."

Before Dr. Julius could suck in his breath so as to let out the blood curdling scream which was just starting to emerge, the lady stood up. Unbelievably, she was even bigger than her son, both taller and heavier. "Louis," she roared. "Put that little man down!" Instead of putting Dr. Julius down, though, the son drew back his fist, which, incidentally, was the size of a ham hock. Instantly, Mrs. Toohey put her head down. Then using it as a battering ram, she ran directly at her son. The force of this huge woman's body knocked him away from Dr. Julius. Feeling himself freed from the clutches of the roaring monster, Dr. Julius ran for the door of the quiet room, threw it open, and took off down the hall. "Call Security!" he yelled, racing down the steps and out of the building. Dr. Julius could really move.

The security guard arrived on the floor just as Big Mama was dragging her howling son onto the elevator. It was a good thing too, since that security guard was all of five feet two and may have weighed a hundred twenty pounds soaking wet. The Tooheys did not return to the hospital. That night the nursing staff did the fastest post mortem care ever known to mankind, and got Mr. Toohey down to the morgue quicker than had ever happened before in that hospital.

When things calmed down, everybody decided that Mr. Toohey's son had just been very upset and most likely never would have hurt Dr. Julius. He was probably like a big bear, they said. Loud, but really not harmful. Dr. Julius, not present at this time may not have been so sure.

Well, two days later, the Big Bear's picture appeared on page one of the newspaper. It seems he had left his father's funeral and had a little run-in with a couple of "friends." After an exchange of some words, he had pulled out a knife and stabbed both of them to death. Too bad Mama Bear wasn't there to prevent it.

So Dr. Julius, when he finally was able to let himself think about what had happened, realized he had come pretty close to becoming a statistic and helping to put his hospital on the map. To this day, every time he has to speak with a family who has just lost someone they love, he thinks about what almost happened that night in the "quiet room."

And he makes sure the door is wide open before he says a word.

Codes

Mr. Kaplan was sixty-two years old and had been diagnosed with lung cancer two years earlier. A very heavy smoker for thirty years, he had given up cigarettes just six months before his harsh persistent cough had indicated the need for a chest x-ray. Mr. Kaplan had lung cancer.

The tumor was removed along with a portion of his lung, and for a while he did very well. Mr. Kaplan enjoyed his second chance at life.

Less than a year after surgery, the cancer was found to have spread to his liver and bones. Bouts of radiation and chemotherapy had slowed the growth of the cancer but now it had spread throughout his body. Mr. Kaplan had lost almost forty pounds and even with the pain medicine, he was always hurting. He was admitted to the oncology floor with the diagnosis of end-stage metastatic lung carcinoma. Mr. Kaplan was somewhat alert and aware of his condition, but he tended to drift in and out of full consciousness.

Dr. Riley was the oncologist in charge of Mr. Kaplan's care. He, the nursing staff and the resident physicians held a conference with the family to discuss their options. Dr. Riley explained that in his opinion, the best and kindest thing that could be done for Mr. Kaplan was to give him large doses of medicine for pain, oxygen to make his breathing less labored, and the tender loving care that oncology nurses are known for, and simply keep Mr. Kaplan comfortable until he died.

The family, however, would not hear of this. They would not stand by and let their husband and father die. They wanted everything possible done. After all, this was a hospital, wasn't it? If it meant tubes and respirators, then that's what they wanted. They had to save him. They loved him too much too let him go, they said.

So Mr. Kaplan's status was listed as a "full code" because that's what the family wanted. Mr. Kaplan was too sick and often too confused to ask what *he* wanted. And, naturally, this was way before the times of living wills and advanced directives. The only concession made by the family was that they would not insist on transferring him to the I.C.U. because they knew all the nurses on the oncology floor and felt more comfortable there.

The next day, while Mr. Kaplan's family was down in the coffee shop, he stopped breathing. Mary, the nursing assistant, had come into the room and found him blue and unresponsive.

84

A cardiac arrest code was called and the team arrived and did its thing. They got his heart started again. But there was just one small problem. Mr. Kaplan had been without oxygen for a period of time that was long enough for a large part of his brain to die.

When Mr. Kaplan's family saw him again, he was in the I.C.U. He had a big tube down his throat which was hooked to a respirator. He had another tube running into a very large vein in the front of his chest through which he was getting lots of big time drugs. The compressions on his chest had caused his cancer-filled bones to crunch and puncture his left lung, and so he needed to have a big hose inserted into the side of his chest to drain the blood and tissue fluid accumulating at the site of the lung laceration. He had a catheter to drain his bladder and a tube in his nose to empty his stomach, alongside the big one coming out of his mouth. To top it off, Mr. Kaplan was having continuous seizures due to the damage to his irritated brain.

"What have you done to my father?" screamed Mr. Kaplan's son. "Stop it! Leave him alone! That's not what we wanted! We just wanted him to get better!"

*****

John had been asthmatic since he was a baby. Now twenty years old, he knew a great deal about his disease and how to take care of himself. For the most part, he led a normal life. He was familiar with the early signs of an asthmatic attack, and knew when to use his inhalers and when he needed medical attention.

He had developed a cold a few days earlier, and was taking antibiotics as prescribed by his doctor. John and his family were aware that asthmatic patients need to prevent full blown respiratory infections, and so he had followed the medical advice exactly.

But for some reason, John became worse. By the time he got to the hospital, he was in real trouble. The respiratory treatments and the intravenous medications didn't help. John couldn't get enough air into his lungs. He was restless and was turning blue. John was sedated so that he wouldn't fight the big tube in his throat, and then he was put on a respirator. He was transferred to the I.C.U.

Well, unlike most similar cases, this standard therapy coupled with potent medications did not combine to open his airways, and John did not improve. He kept getting worse. Then, two hours after his admission to the intensive care unit, his heartbeat suddenly dropped to a rate of about twenty per minutes and then stopped completely. John was clinically dead. A cardiac arrest code was called.

John's parents and sisters, out in the waiting room, heard the call and knew that something horrible had happened. Someone went to sit with them. Within five minutes John's heart began to beat normally. At first it wasn't possible to see if John was O.K.

ntally, since along with the heavy sedation, he had been receiving medication to ralyze his entire body. So the wait began for the drugs to wear off. It was a very ng hour. Then John opened his eyes and nodded in response to questions. He was e!

Ten days later, John was discharged from the hospital, once again happy and althy. Thankfully, he had absolutely no memory of anything from the time he came to the emergency room until he was transferred to the regular medical floor.

*****

So what happened here? Isn't it true that a code is a code is a code? Uh, uh. ope. Ask any hospital nurse. It doesn't work that way. Reviving a dying heart in a ring body, is wrong, as almost all these nurses will agree. C.P.R. is to save someone's e, to prolong their living and not their dying.

Cardiac arrest codes are completely gray issues, though, and not black and white es. Who's to say that one person should live and another is ready to die? Even spital ethics committees may disagree on what should happen.

And what about these "slow codes", where teams go through the motions of suscitation without really trying? This type of code is usually due to family pressures hen the staff agrees that there is "nothing left to save." And "chemical codes" are a ke. Potent code drugs like adrenalin and atropine are given, but C.P.R. is not rformed. So what happens to these "chemicals"? Once the heart stops, the drugs n't do anything but sit in the vein. They don't circulate anywhere. So what's the int?

Then there are those crazy directives like, "Do C.P.R. but do not intubate." This eans try, but don't try everything because the patient may end up on a respirator, and at shouldn't happen. The same goes for, "Do C.P.R. but do not defibrillate." That tle gem usually means that the family says to try to save the patient but they don't want m "electric shocked." Come on.

And last but not least comes the old "coffee code." This is most often an nwritten directive which in effect tells the staff that if they find the patient without a lse or respiratory effort, they should go have a nice hot cup of coffee before they call e code. By that time, then, they will have done what the family wanted, but with no ance of reviving the patient. Cute.

The power of our life and death decisions is truly awesome. We've come a long ay, baby. But boy, oh boy, do we have along way to go!

All In A Day's Work

(Yes, it's a poem!)

It's seven o'clock in the morning,
There's more staff than you've had in a while.
You've got nurses and aides
To cover your floor,
You look at each other and smile.

And then the phone rings,
You know what that brings,
"Oh, no!" you hear everyone say.
"We must pull," says the voice,
"Send Jenny or Joyce,
They need help on 6-West right away!"

It's six o'clock in the evening,
You're finally ready to eat.
In walks Dr. Geddy,
"Hi, girls! Are you ready?
What's wrong? You look kind of beat!"

"Let's do this procedure,
I'm going to need ya,
To help me, so let's get a start.
I need you to set up,
Raise Mr. Smith's bed up.
I'm putting a Swan in his heart."

It's five o'clock on the night shift,
The unit is starting to hush,
The patients are sleeping,
Supplies are away,
It looks like there's no need to rush.

Then out of the blue.
You hear "Code 22!"
And everyone jumps to their feet.
You know now you blew it,
You never should do it.
Don't think that you've got the shift beat!

"All In A Day's Work," by Linda Strangio, RN, MA, CCRN. From: **Nursing Spectrum,** New York/ New Jersey Metro Edition. Reprinted with permission.

Detective Hanrahan

It had turned into a really messy situation. Jenny had been extremely sloppy with her use and documentation of narcotics and other controlled drugs, and the investigation had been long and involved.

But Jenny had denied any wrongdoing, and there had been lots of anger and tears. As it stood now, she was on probation until the matter was resolved and the Board of Nursing had temporarily suspended her license. The nurses all were heartbroken, since they had known Jennie a long time. It really hurt.

So the staff was told not to discuss the matter with anyone. It was to be kept strictly confidential. Any communication was going to be done officially through the hospital administration. If there was to be any more questioning of anyone, the powers that be were to be involved. That matter was made perfectly clear.

Kathryn was the nurse who had worked the closest with Jennie for the longest time. She felt the worst. Even though they had never really become friends, Kathryn and Jennie routinely ate their dinner together and did their evening bedside nursing care as a team.

It was a quiet spring evening, Kathryn's day off. She had taken it easy that day, done a little shopping and read a bit. Kathryn was in her kitchen, washing the dishes and planning to flop down and watch some television, when her phone rang.

"Hello," answered Kathryn. "This is Detective Hanrahan of the Federal Narcotics Bureau," the voice on the other end tersely announced. "We need to come over to your house right away to discuss some very sensitive information we have just learned regarding the actions of Jennie Glover. It is you who have been working closely with Miss Glover, have you not?" the voice questioned.

Kathryn hesitated. Her instructions had been quite clear. But this was now something big time. She didn't know what to say. "Well," Kathryn replied. "Yes, I worked with Jennie, but my administration has told me not to discuss the matter with anyone."

"Look here, Miss," the detective responded, a hint of anger in his voice. "This is federal business, and you would be wise to realize that our office overrules any instructions you may have received. This matter cannot wait, and if you do not cooperate with us, you may be obstructing justice. Think about that before you refuse."

Kathryn felt a knot forming in the bottom of her stomach. "O.K.," she said in a little voice. "I guess you can come over. Do you know where I live?" The voice laughed. "Of course, we do. We'll be over in about twenty minutes." And then Detective Hanrahan hung up.

Well, Kathryn started getting more and more scared. What should she say to these people? Should she tell them everything she knew? She'd gone over and over the information with the hospital people and they should really be the ones to speak to the Narcotic Bureau, not her. In fact, she was almost certain that the hospital administrators had been in touch with them already. What had her hospital done, given her name to the Feds? Maybe they thought she was an accomplice or something.

By this time, Kathryn was on the verge of panic. She didn't know what to do, so she started to scream at her husband that federal agents were on their way over. She had visions of herself being dragged off in handcuffs with her kids screaming in the background and all the neighbors standing outside gawking at her. Oh, God, what should she do?

So Kathryn ran to the phone and called the evening supervisor. Naturally it had to be Mrs. McLaughlin who was working. Mrs. McLaughlin usually was even more emotional than Kathryn. And considering Kathryn's usual mental state, that had to be pretty wild. Kathryn told Mrs. McLaughlin, or rather babbled to her, what had happened. And as could be expected, Mrs. McLaughlin became very upset. She always needed to do things by the book, and in a case like this, she had no book to follow.

"Now, listen, Mrs. Boone," said Mrs. McLaughlin. (Mrs. McLaughlin always called everyone by their last names.) "Don't you speak to these people until I get back to you. I am going to call Mrs. Drummond for instructions. Don't even let them in the door."

Kathryn groaned. She had a vision of barricading the front door while these federal agents were trying to get inside. That would look really great for her; no doubt they would assume she had progressed from an accomplice to narcotic theft to mass murder or something like that. Mrs. Drummond was the Director of Nursing, and now it had gone up to that level. What next?

Well, Kathryn didn't have to wonder very long. Within five minutes Mrs. Drummond called her back, and she seemed extremely concerned about what was going on. "Listen to me, Kathryn," she said tensely. "I'm not quite sure what has happened with this case, but I really have no idea why the Narcotic Bureau needs to question you at home tonight. I have decided to bring this directly to Mr. Liberto. I want you to wait by the phone. I will call him and get right back to you." Then Mrs. Drummond hung up the phone.

By now Kathryn was an absolute wreck. Mr. Liberto was the President and C.E.O. of the whole hospital. My God, Kathryn whimpered to herself. What is going to happen now?

As soon as Kathryn hung up the phone, it rang. It was her best friend, Jackie, also a nurse in their unit. "Well, hi, hon!" announced Jackie cheerfully. "What's new?" Kathryn started to scream like a maniac. "Get off the phone!" she shrieked wildly. "I'm waiting for Mrs. Drummond or Mr. Liberto to call me back!"

There was silence for a minute and then Jackie asked very quietly, "Uh, Kathryn, why would Mrs. Drummond or Mr. Liberto be calling you?" Kathryn yelled into the phone like a wild woman. "The Federal Narcotic Bureau is coming over to talk to me about Jennie! I can't believe all this is happening to me! They probably think I was stealing drugs with her! I'm so scared, Jackie! I called the hospital and nobody knows what to do! We're waiting for instructions from Mr. Liberto!"

Now there was an even longer silence. Then Jackie spoke. Softly - very softly - she asked, "Um, Kathryn, was the person who called you named Detective Hanrahan?" For a minute, Kathryn was blank. "Yes, she said," slowly. "How did you know?"

"Now, Kathryn," Jackie said quietly. "Please don't go crazy, but that wasn't a real detective. That was my husband, Jim. It was an April Fool joke, Kathryn. Today is April Fools Day, remember?"

For a few seconds Kathryn was silent, and then suddenly she lost it. She started to scream and cry. "I can't believe you did this to me! Now, I'm going to get fired! I thought you were my friend! Oh, I'll never forgive you for this!" Jackie started to scream also. "Don't yell at me," she said. "It's your fault for being so stupid and forgetting it's April Fools Day! Most normal people, even if they had believed the whole thing, would have run around and straightened up the house. They wouldn't have started making crazy phone calls to everyone. Oh, I'm surprised you didn't call the Governor or the President of the United States!" At that point they both slammed the phone down.

By this time, Kathryn was crying quietly. What on earth would she say when Mrs. Drummond or Mr. Liberto called her back? Kathryn's husband was pacing around the living room bellowing things like, "What kind of mental cases do you have for friends?"

Within a few minutes, the phone rang again. Kathryn, her hands shaking, picked it up. "Hello," she said in a tiny little voice. It was Mrs. Drummond. "Kathryn," the Director of Nursing said tensely. "I just spoke to Mr. Liberto, and this is what we want you to say."

"Oh, Mrs. Drummond," whimpered Kathryn into the phone. "You'll never guess what just happened. The same voice who said he was Detective Hanrahan just called back. He said to me, 'This is Detective Hanrahan. April Fool.' And then he hung up the phone. I guess the whole think was an April Fools joke. Isn't that something, Mrs. Drummond?" And with that Kathryn started to giggle hysterically.

There was an audible sigh on Mrs. Drummond's end. Then dead silence. "Alright, Kathryn," she said slowly and quietly. "Good night." And that was that.

Well, it took a week or two but finally Kathryn was able to speak to her best friend Jackie again. They made a pact never to tell anybody what really happened that night, because they were quite sure that if the truth got out, they would both be unemployed. Mrs. McLaughlin asked Kathryn if she knew who played the prank, and of course Kathryn said that she had no idea. But they both knew that was a big fat lie.

And every year when April first comes close, Kathryn and Jackie think back to that crazy evening when Detective Hanrahan made his famous phone call. Now, it seems sort of funny.

Three Ladies

Lady number one was brought into the emergency room by her daughter. Her pain was in her abdomen, and as she put it, it went "right through to her back." Besides the pain, Mrs. Jameson suddenly couldn't stand up; her legs had become very weak. But other than that, she didn't feel so terrible. In fact, she was getting hungry. Well, Mrs. Jameson was brought over to the CT department to see what was going on, and sure enough, she was in trouble. Big trouble.

Her aorta had a huge aneurysm, which was in the process of dissecting. It could be seen right there on the screen. What the CT scan also showed was a kidney which had already died due to lack of blood supply. And the same thing had happened to a section of her spinal cord. No wonder she had trouble standing up.

By the time the pictures were completed, the emergency room physician, a neurologist, and a vascular surgeon were all present in the scanning room. Even a young person would most probably die on the operating room table, and this lady was eighty-six years old.

So the three doctors walked back to the emergency department together to talk to the patient and her family and explain what was going on. A half hour later, Mrs. Jameson was upstairs in a regular room, with her family at her bedside. She had asked for a cup of coffee and an English muffin with grape jelly. They wanted to give her a steak. Maybe filet mignon. But all she wanted was that coffee and the muffin. So it was brought to her right away and she enjoyed every bit of it, even though her abdomen was starting to become quite distended with blood. By this time, the morphine drip had taken over and Mrs. Jameson drifted off into a pain-free sleep. Her abdomen continued to grow until her heart finally stopped pumping blood out of her leaking circulatory system.

The very next day, Mrs. McNeill came in to the same emergency room with the same type of symptoms. She also was thought to have a dissecting aortic aneurysm. It couldn't be, thought the staff. This lady was the same age as Mrs. Jameson. In fact, they even looked alike.

But there was the dissection, unmistakable on the CT screen. While still on the table, she told the staff that she had had a great time the day before. She had taken a bus trip to Atlantic City, she said with a smile, and had returned with a hundred fifty dollars of Donald Trump's money. She had been so lucky, she thought, that maybe her luck would hold through the operation. She wanted to take the chance.

So lady number two went off to the operating room where the operating team tried everything they could to patch this lady's aorta and save her life. But Mrs. McNeill's luck had run out along with all her clotting factors. Three hours after the surgery began, Mrs. McNeill bled to death.

That same afternoon, lady number three came into the emergency department with the same complaints as Mrs. Jameson and Mrs. McNeill. She was sent to the CT department with the same working diagnosis, and sure enough, there it was on the CT screen: a big aortic aneurysm which was beginning to leak. Mrs. Whitman was certain that the only reason her back hurt so much was the fact that she had to lie on that hard scanning table. It took a while until she understood what was happening to her. Like Mrs. McNeill, she wanted the operation.

Well, this time the staff had a good feeling, a feeling that this lady would beat the odds of surviving a true leaking aortic aneurysm. And she did. Mrs. Whitman was brought up to the intensive care unit with good vital signs, excellent pressure readings, and a great urinary output. The next morning Mrs. Whitman was out of bed in the chair and watching television. She did great.

Three ladies. Three elderly, happy ladies.

All had full lives and all were healthy up until the day their aneurysms, which they never knew they had, blew. But lady number one had died peacefully in her bed. Her wishes had been followed, and she was allow to die quickly and painlessly. Lady number two died the day following one of the best in her life. She went into a deep sleep in the operating room and just never woke up. And lady number three, who made it, was back at home with her family within a few short weeks.

Not a bad ending for any of them.

The Day From Hell

It was the worst of days, one of the most horrible they could ever remember. The staffing was lousy, the patients were totally unstable, and the phones never stopped. Everything went wrong. Patients had trouble breathing, dropped their blood pressures, and developed dangerous cardiac rhythms. For an I.C.U. where out of the ordinary events were ordinary, this day was something else.

From the minute the day staff walked in, they knew they were doomed. All nurses know the mood and what it means. Nobody has to say a word. The unit was a wreck. In front of the nurses' station was the crash cart, open and almost totally depleted. The laundry bags were overflowing and the desk was piled high with charts and clipboards. Call lights were flashing and the alarm bells on the intravenous infusion pumps were ringing away. Reams of paper were hanging from the cardiac monitor banks, showing that alarms had been signaling problems.

Only one of the day nurses had a set of clean scrubs in her locker. And the cart which normally kept them was empty, except for one top - a pair of 3 XX. Naturally. Not having any time to run to the O.R. to grab green scrubs, the staff began to take report in their street clothes. One of the nurses put the jumbo giant top on over her jeans, and as would be expected, she looked totally ridiculous. But nobody cared. They needed to get started.

The night staff was almost two hours late getting off, since there was so much catching up to do. By the time they had given report and finished up their charts, they were not only thoroughly exhausted but totally disgusted. And by then, the day from hell was well under way for the day nurses.

Nobody ate or even got a chance to gulp a cup of coffee that day. The head nurse on that unit always told them they had to stop to eat, since "they couldn't take care of their patients until they first took care of themselves." Very nice. Very cute. However, she was not at work this particular day and they were. She had taken a vacation day and was probably still in her comfortable warm bed or out shopping somewhere.

At eleven o'clock, they got an order to take Mrs. Rafferty down to C.T. Scan. Mrs. Rafferty was probably the sickest patient in the unit, and was what the staff called a "train wreck." If you could name a tube, she had it. If you could think of a medication, she was on it. She was like a big water balloon, and must have been carrying a hundred pounds of fluid which weeped out through her skin which had the consistency of tissue paper. Whenever she was removed from the ventilator, even for a few seconds, she turned blue. Mrs. Rafferty could barely tolerate being turned, and her trips to the hemodialysis unit were total fiascos. And now she had to go to Radiology which wasn't even in the same building.

A half hour after the time they were supposed to be downstairs, the C.T. department called. Yes, they understood what it meant to transport a patient like Mrs. Rafferty, and yes, they knew how many people were involved in the move, and yes, they knew that like all the areas in the hospital the staffing was bad, BUT--they needed Mrs. Rafferty *right now* because their schedule was packed and they couldn't hold the table open any more. SO HURRY UP! The nurses wanted to scream.

The move to C.T. scan and back was something else. It took about six people to push her and all her equipment. Even with steady bagging, she looked like she was about to code by the time she arrived there, and after finally dragging her onto the table everyone was physically and mentally drained. The scan lasted only ten minutes, and in the opinion of everyone, was not necessary. The nurses just wished there would be some kind of a rule that the doctor who ordered these ridiculous "road trips" needed to take part in them.

There were nine people present as Mrs. Rafferty was pulled off the scanning table and somehow, someway, her triple lumen catheter still managed to slide right out of her jugular vein. Nobody even said a word. They just shook their heads and sighed. When the staff and Mrs. Rafferty arrived back in the unit, there was a patient lying on the floor. She had fallen out of bed while trying to get up to go to the bathroom, since nobody had come to answer her call light. And why hadn't anyone come? Because almost everyone had left the unit for the big travel adventure.

None of the patients had gotten morning care yet, and by this time it was afternoon. Mr. McQueen started to scream at that point, and when one of the nurses went in to check him she found him covered with diarrhea. It oozed up to his shoulders and dripped down to his calves. And it stank. Poor Mr. McQueen. It was obvious that every time he had a bowel movement, he suffered terrible cramps. And the stuff most likely burned his already excoriated skin. So cleaning Mr. McQueen became the priority, but also took two nurses. Twenty minutes later, he was all clean and covered with sweet smelling body lotion. The stinky sheets had been replaced with fresh clean ones and the dirty linen hamper emptied. As the nurses breathed a sigh of relief, Mr. McQueen began to scream again. Oh, no, the nurses thought as they stared soundlessly at each other. Oh, yes. This time it was up past the pillow and down to his toes.

By then it was time for the visitors to come in. And then the complaints started. Their mothers (fathers, sisters, husbands, wives) were too hot, too cold, hungry, thirsty,

96

in pain, needed to turn, to sit up, to lie down, wanted another blanket, some ice chips, some water, a glass of tea, etc., etc. They needed bedpans, their teeth brushed, their hair combed, and so on. Meanwhile, the nurses were two hours behind in their medications, I.V.'s were running dry, vital signs and pressures were not recorded, and all the STAT things the patients needed hadn't been done yet. The emergency department had patients to be admitted and of course the I.C.U. was full. There were no orders to transfer and no priorities, since nobody had any time to get them. It was simply horrible.

Suddenly, right in the middle of this nightmare, appeared the patient from hell. Mr. LoPresto had bolted from his room, ripping off his gown and pulling out almost all his tubes. He stood there in the middle of the unit, naked as a jaybird except for the foley catheter which protruded from his penis, still attached to the drainage bag which trailed behind him on the floor. Blood dripped from the sites where his three I.V. bags had once infused fluids and drugs into his body. Green bile, which had leaked from the nasogastric tube as he had snatched it out of his nose, covered his chest and upper abdomen. He somehow had overlooked his Udall dialysis catheter which dangled precariously out of his right groin. One monitor lead with its snaky black cable hung from his right shoulder.

Wild eyed, Mr.LoPresto roared, "I'm getting out of this prison! They're trying to kill me! Get the cops!" And with that he started to run up and down the unit, dripping blood and dragging his foley bag with him. Oh, yes, and Mr. LoPresto also just happened to have a virulent strain of active tuberculosis, and had been on strict respiratory isolation in a private reverse laminar flow isolation room. In addition, Mr.LoPresto was over six feet tall and weighed more than three hundred pounds, and he looked like a linebacker as he ran the length of the corridor. The seclusion team, which was paged overhead, had a hard time handling Mr. Lopresto, and of course all the visitors had a birds' eye view of this entire charming scene.

By the time Mr. LoPresto was restrained back in his bed and most of his tubes replaced, the nursing staff had just about had it. Nobody knew where to start, to try to begin to get things together. And it was at that exact moment that a visitor approached the desk. She was a prissy, prim, holier than thou, pain in the butt, know it all, perfectly dressed middle aged lady. And comparing her to the motley group of wild eyed exhausted women wearing patient gowns over their street clothes, she looked even more impeccable. "Excuse me," she said loudly to the group of nurses. "Would you mind explaining to me just how you people allowed this to happen?"

There was no sound for a minute as the nurses tried to control themselves. A little moan escaped through the lips of one of them, as the second nurse turned her back and walked away. With a straight face, the first nurse then simply said, "Why, we encourage it. We thoroughly enjoy this." And with that she left the nurses' station, knowing full well that something was going to be made of this. Oh, yes, she was sure she would be hearing from the nursing office about her "rude manner" and "lack of professionalism." That perfect little lady would see to it.

But right then and right there, she honestly could care less. Only another nurse could understand the situation. The visitor from hell coupled with the patient from hell topped off the unit from hell to round out the day from hell.

And it was far from over.

Good Judgement

1. Mrs. Jackson had just been admitted with the diagnosis of "acute abdomen." Aside from a little belly pain, she actually looked pretty good. "I just don't know why some of these patients are admitted," sighed Mary Beth. "And I really don't understand why they even come to the emergency room. Take Mrs. Jackson, for example. I'm sure there's nothing wrong with her." Mary Beth went in to admit Mrs. Jackson to the unit. "Let me put your mind at ease," Mary Beth told her patient. "I've been a nurse for a lot of years, and I am almost positive that by tomorrow you'll be completely better. You probably just have gas pains." Mrs. Jackson smiled, looking visibly relieved.

Follow-up - That night Mrs. Jackson was taken to the operating room. She had a ruptured diverticulum and ended up with a colostomy.

2. Mr. O'Neal was over in Nuclear Medicine having a bleeding scan. Phyllis hated those exams because they lasted up to five hours. And if they found an active bleeding site, the patients usually were brought over to Special Procedures for an abdominal angiogram. "This man looks better than you do, Phyllis said to John. In fact, I'm so sure the scan will be negative that I can tell you that I will eat this x-ray table if it isn't."

Follow-up - An hour later Phyllis got a phone call from Nuclear Medicine. "Come to Room 10," the voice said, "and bring your salt shaker." Mr. O'Neal is bleeding into his right colon."

3. Tom had been in a car accident and had been moderately confused for several weeks. Today he was perfectly lucid, saying he remembered nothing about what had happened. He seemed fine to Marion, who was leaving at the end of her evening shift. "I left him unrestrained," Marion told Toni. "There's absolutely no reason to tie his hands. He's fine." "Marion," warned Toni. "If he pulls anything out tonight, I'll kill you. We're working short staffed and I can't be babysitting for Tom." Marion laughed. "Believe me, Toni," she said reassuringly. "He's perfectly alert."

Follow-up - When Marion got out of the shower at home about an hour later, the phone was ringing. It was Toni. "I should make you come back to work and put all these tubes back," said Toni with a sigh. "I'm calling to let you know that Tom just pulled out his I.V., his feeding tube and his foley. Thanks for your insight."

By The Dawn's Early Light

Annette always dressed up for the holidays. At Easter time, she wore bunnies and ducks, and at Thanksgiving she came to work decked out with turkeys and Pilgrims all over her. She was practically a walking Christmas tree in December. The patients got a kick out of seeing all of this, and Annette loved it when she saw how it made them smile, sick as they might be. Now it was the week before Halloween, one of her favorite times. She varied her costumes, and today she had a large monster pin attached to the front of her scrubs, complete with a battery which triggered loud horror music when it was pressed.

In the half-light of the early morning, Annette leaned over Mrs. Kennedy's bed. The lady had come up from the Recovery Room just nine hours earlier, after having most of her stomach and esophagus removed. She was intubated and on a ventilator. She had a pulmonary artery catheter through which several drips were infusing, as well as a peripheral I.V. site. An arterial line was in place, as was a foley catheter. An epidural catheter was taped to her back and shoulder, and her nasogastric tube was sutured in place. The cardiac monitor cable was draped across her chest, and various numbers and waveforms beeped and flashed across the screens. Her hands were restrained. Talk about sensory bombardment!

Even with her sedation, Mrs. Kennedy was awake and appeared to be terrified. As Annette opened her mouth to utter soft words of reassurance, the front of her monster pin hit the side rail of the I.C.U. bed. Loud eerie music suddenly blared forth. Mrs. Kennedy, unable to speak, opened her eyes wide in horror. She strained at her tubes and restraints, trying to break free.

Oh, my God, thought Annette, as she leaned over Mrs. Kennedy's bed. This poor lady, who most likely has no memory of what has happened to her, now probably thinks she has died and is in hell. Annette didn't know whether to laugh or cry.

Doctor Potato Head

His real name was Dr. Peter Corliss, but the nurses called him Dr. Potato Head. He looked like Mr. Potato Head, that plastic toy potato with slits for the arms and legs. Dr. Corliss had a big head which sort of came to a point on top. Just like Mr. Potato Head.

Now, nobody would ever have started calling Dr. Corliss Dr. Potato Head if he had been a different person. The overwhelming majority of the doctors got along just fine with the nurses. Each treated the other with friendship and respect. But Dr. Potato Head was not part of that overwhelming majority. He, in fact, never spoke to a nurse unless he needed something. If he passed a nurse in the hall, he ignored her. Or more likely, he probably never even noticed her. If a nurse said hello to Dr. Potato Head, he looked blankly at her as if she were a ghost. He spoke to the doctors all the time. But not to the nurses.

Dr. Potato Head was an internist. He was never blatantly rude or arrogant to nurses. He just believed that whatever it was they were doing, it wasn't as important as his needs. For example, if a group of nurses were speaking to each other or a nurse was on the phone, Dr. Potato Head would chime right in with whatever it was he wanted. He interrupted them because he obviously believed that was the way it should be. And he always called them "girls." It didn't matter if the nurse was twenty-one or sixty-one, she was a "girl." "Girls, I need Mr. Brown's chart," he'd yell while two nurses were turning a patient. Or during report, he'd interrupt by calling out loud, "Girls, was Mrs. Jones' lung scan done today?" He never spoke to the male nurses, probably because he had no clue who they were. And he probably didn't care.

Well, one particular evening, all this changed. It was close to nine o'clock and the three nurses were doing their charts at the nurses' station. For a change, the phones weren't ringing and nobody else was at the desk. The floor was very quiet.

Suddenly Dr. Potato Head strode onto the floor. He walked into the nurses' station and past the three nurses. Opening the door of the little staff bathroom right behind the main desk, he walked in and closed the door. That bathroom was probably the least private in the whole hospital, and nobody ever used it except to wash their hands. The nurses looked at each other, and before they could even start to make faces, sounds started to erupt from that bathroom. Obviously, Dr. Potato Head had a belly ache or something, because the gas emerging from him sounded as if it was enough to blow up more than a few balloons. And those sound effects lasted a very long time.

The three nurses stared at each other, wild-eyed, trying not to laugh out loud. Two of them clamped their hands over their mouths. The third got up and ran into the medication room. The sounds continued for a while, along with several flushes of the toilet bowl. By the time the nurses heard the water running in the sink, they had gotten themselves back under control.

As Dr. Potato Head opened the door of the little bathroom, he seemed to suddenly become aware of the people sitting just a few feet away. Maybe it was because all of them must have had some type of little smirk on their faces, or perhaps he realized just how close the toilet seat he had been sitting on was from his audience. Either way, Dr. Potato Head's pointy face turned red. His eyes darted from one nurse to the other and then he looked down at the floor. "Girls," he announced, to nobody in particular. And then he quickly left the unit.

Well, after that night it seemed that Dr. Potato Head began to notice people other than physicians. He actually looked at the nurses as he spoke to them. Maybe it was because he was embarrassed and wanted to be sure that none of them were those whom he serenaded late that evening.

Oh, and Dr. Potato Head got another name. Dr. Peter Corliss became known as Dr. Fart.

A Pain in the Neck

He didn't even know he was hurt, but the next day he had a vague memory of falling backwards off a front step. His neck was a little sore, though, and he had kind of a tingling in his arm. Nothing big.

George had often done things that he didn't quite remember, since George was often drunk. Very drunk. He spent his time with his cronies who lived just as he did. They all seemed to be happy, although they were not exactly in the best of health. At least by other people's standards.

But George was content with his life. What he did with it, by the way, was really not very much. He and his pals spent their time talking, playing cards, and drinking beer and wine. George was a nice person, happy go lucky, and friendly to everyone. He was a nice guy.

Nobody seemed to remember exactly why George came to the emergency room that next day. As many people do, George used the E.R. as a walk-in doctor's office for whatever ailed him. Colds, headaches, etc. - - - that's where he got his cough medicine and his pain medicine. But this time was different. Maybe the funny feeling in his arm bothered him a little.

While he was there, George casually mentioned that he had fallen and bruised his neck. There was, in fact, a bit of a discoloration and swelling, and the area was tender to the touch. So off George went for x-rays, and the results shocked everyone. It seems that George had a severe fracture and dislocation of two of the vertebrae in his neck. And they were starting to compress, just a tiny bit, George's spinal cord.

Well, this was big stuff. If not immobilized immediately, George could become a quadriplegic. Something had to be done right away. So George went off to the intensive care unit to be put into traction. Now this was well before halo vests came into being, and the way that cervical fractures or subluxations were treated was by inserting tongs into the sides of the head, attaching weights to the tongs, and then keeping the patient on a turning frame for about twelve weeks. That was the way the traction was maintained. So for about three full months patients were kept immobile, either flat on their backs or on prone on their stomachs. This was a bad time in medical history to break one's neck. Very uncomfortable.

George seemed to understand the whats and whys and hows of the treatment. At least he said he did. But George, being a friendly guy, always seemed to agree with everything and everyone. "O.K.," he said. "Do what you have to do."

By that afternoon, George was on the frame with his neck just the way they wanted it. Aside from some soreness at the site of the tongs insertion, he didn't appear to be very uncomfortable. He fell asleep on his back and stayed that way for a few hours. The nurses, knowing how hard it is for some patients to tolerate this type of long term therapy, were relieved. They were glad that George was such an easygoing guy.

Yeah, right.

When George finally woke up, he seemed to be a bit restless. He tried to sit up, and when he couldn't, he began to scream. The nurses tried to calm George and repeated and reinforced everything that had been said to him. When they asked him if he understood that he could only lie flat and not move his head, he said he did. But within ten minutes, George was once again trying to sit straight up. And screaming.

And that began the horror of the next few months, days which stretched into long weeks, during which a constant battle played out between the nurses and the patient. A battle in which the goal of the nursing staff was to keep the patient from getting loose from those tongs and permanently damaging his spinal cord. And a battle in which the goal of the patient was to get off that frame and get moving.

Now if all of this was taking place today, things probably would be a bit different. There would be psychiatrists involved to declare competency, ethics committees would meet, and all of the other stuff involving patients and their rights would come into play. But back then, the doctors and the hospitals were in charge. Nobody worried about lawsuits or unlawful imprisonment charges or anything like that. So George was kept on that frame. And he didn't like it one bit.

Of course George went through his share of alcohol withdrawal. He got lots of librium to try to calm him, but apparently it wasn't enough. He yelled and carried on those first few days, and continuously tried to get up off that turning frame. The nurses were scared to death that he was going to rip those tongs out of his skull and throw himself on the floor. Then, they were sure, there would be instant paralysis and maybe even death.

So every time George started to thrash around, someone would go racing into his room to try to calm him down. The neurosurgeon wasn't much help to the staff. Each time they tried to get George's sedation increased, the doctor came out with little digs like, "Well, if you nurses gave him some old fashioned T.L.C., he wouldn't need any sedation at all." He was a real pip, that guy.

Many times a nurse passed George's room to find that he had squirmed off the side of the frame and was literally hanging by his tongs. Everyone became nervous wrecks waiting for the inevitable. It got so bad that whenever George woke up and started to get restless, the staff would sandwich him between the two frames just to hold him in place. It looked and sounded like a torture chamber in there. George howled constantly.

Nobody knew for sure if George had totally flipped out or if he just wanted to get out of there, no matter what the consequences. Many times he was totally lucid, but within short periods he seemed completely irrational. "George, lie still! You're going to kill yourself," were the words heard most often during those days. The only time the nurses were calm was when George was sleeping deeply.

Well, somehow, twelve weeks passed. It was time to get George up off the frame. The nurses were ecstatic, probably more so than George. The stress involved with the possibility of George falling off the frame was over. Finally. But testing showed that George's neck was far from stable. That surprised nobody, since everyone knew that the traction had not been properly maintained. It was a miracle, they said, that it hadn't done any more damage to those vertebrae, which had taken the weight of George's acrobatic stunts.

There was no doubt that he would never keep a big heavy Philadelphia collar in place, so George was put into a crazy looking plaster cast. It covered his chest and went up his neck and framed his head in order to keep it from moving. The nurses laughed because the spica cast really looked like a white plaster halo. And George was far being an angel.

George was thrilled to be able to be up and walking. He turned back into a sweet lovable man again, telling the nurses he knew he had been a pain in the neck. That was really funny because that was the reason for all his trouble. A pain in his neck. Well, George was finally sent home in his big plaster cast and told to take it easy. Everyone breathed a big sigh of relief.

When George came to the clinic ten days later, he no longer looked like an angel. He had managed to break the cast in half and throw away the part that "bothered him." George appeared wearing the plaster vest on his chest and nothing else. From the top of his chest there was no cast. It was gone. He told everyone that it kept him from turning his head and was very annoying. All smiles, he announced that he felt so much better this way. He was his original charming self, smelling like alcohol and sweat. And x-rays showed the bones in his neck to be exactly the way they were on day one. Nothing was healed.

So they just gave up. The remainder of the plaster cast was cut off his chest and everyone documented everything and George was discharged from the clinic. It just wasn't meant for George to be paralyzed, the staff decided. By all reasoning, he should be a quadriplegic or dead, but he was perfectly fine.

George died about five years later, from an unrelated cause. And during that time he functioned just fine with his broken neck. No problems at all.

Get The Head! The Stretcher's Coming!

The fact that Andrea still remembers all the details really amazes her. After all, it happened when she was a student nurse and that was about a zillion years ago.

Back then, nursing school was different. Students were used for service to their hospitals, and were expected to staff the floors as they "learned." That was then what today is known as clinical experience.

This was day two of her obstetrical experience. O.B. rotation consisted of two months in the maternity department, and the time was broken up into labor and delivery, post-partum, nursery, and clinic. The students had full patient assignments back then; they didn't have any time for plain old observation.

That morning Andrea was assigned to a patient in labor. She was a "grand multip", getting ready to have her eighth child. Now in those "good old days", everyone was heavily sedated when they went into labor and put to sleep when they delivered. There was no natural childbirth or anything like that. Women were knocked out and kept in the labor room until they were ready to deliver, and then they were wheeled in to the combination delivery - operating room where they had the baby. If anything went wrong, they were all set up to do the C-Section, and the patient was none the wiser until she woke up from anesthesia. It was a lot easier that way, they believed. At least for the staff. Nobody needed to deal with those minor annoyances like husbands, families, and the miracle of birth itself.

So here was this lady, so knocked out from her drugs that she was really totally unresponsive to everything. And to top it off, her labor was being induced. Now, back then there were no such things as infusion pumps for I.V.'s, or anything remotely similar to control or monitor flow rates. The pitocin was in an I.V. bottle, just running at a "keep vein open" rate. Andrea was sitting alone in the labor room with her patient. Both of them were doing absolutely nothing. Andrea was just there, staring at Mrs. Castaldo's face. If she was supposed to be timing contractions or something like that, she didn't know it. The head nurse had just brought her into the labor room, told her that was her patient for the day, and left. Nothing else. And Mrs. Castaldo seemed to be just fast asleep, not having any labor pains or anything.

A few minutes later, the attending obstetrician came into the room. He gave Andrea a cheery hello and did the same to Mrs. Castaldo. Mrs. Castaldo, of course, did not answer him. The doctor proceeded to do a quick exam and said out loud, "Let's get

some contractions going here!" With that, he opened up the clamp on the I.V. tubi
and the pitocin started to fly into Mrs. Castaldo's vein. He then turned and left the lab
room.

Now Andrea, who had no idea if she was supposed to do anything except sit a
stare at Mrs. Castaldo, began to feel a few uneasy twinges. Is something supposed
happen now, she wondered? She wanted to go out to ask one of the nurses, but s
knew she wasn't supposed to leave her patient. So she continued to sit there with h
eyes glued to Mrs. Castaldo's face. Later she realized that maybe that wasn't the part
the anatomy she should have been watching.

About five minutes later, Mrs. Castaldo started to move around in the bed a
moan a little. But her eyes were still tightly shut, and whatever she was doing, she w
still doing it in her sleep. At this point, Andrea knew that something was changing. SI
got up enough courage to stand up and peek under the sheets. She saw a little bit
blood. Hmmnn, she said to herself. We just learned in class that increased restlessne
and increased bloody show are signs of impending delivery in a multip. And this lac
had already delivered seven kids. But this can't be, she reminded herself. The doct
had examined her just a few minutes ago and said she wasn't doing anything.

Well, five seconds after those words of wisdom popped into Andrea's mind,
bright blue head emerged from between Mrs. Castaldo's legs. The head stopped. Ju
stopped. It didn't keep coming out, and it didn't seem to be attached to a body. It ju
stopped there. And boy, was it blue!

Andrea could not move. She just froze. She couldn't speak or call for help or r
to the door. She just stood there like a statue, transfixed with what she was seeing. A
that exact moment, the labor room door flew open, and in strode the obstetrician with
newspaper in his hand. He was reading it. "Well, young lady," he jovially aske
Andrea. "How's my girl doing?"

"Uh, duhh," brilliantly mumbled Andrea. "The head is out."

The doctor went nuts. He threw the newspaper across the room, screaming
the top of his lungs at Andrea. "You goddamn jackass!" he yelled. "You're ju
standing there doing nothing and letting my patient have her baby alone. What the he
is wrong with you, you moron!" he hollered at her. With that he turned on his heel ar
left the labor room.

Well, Andrea suddenly came to life and sprang into action. She threw the doc
open which went between the labor room she was in and the one her friend Laurie w
in next door. Laurie was sitting there staring at her own sedated patient. "Get the hea
Laurie," she screamed. "The stretcher's coming!" Laurie just looked at her blankly as
Andrea had totally lost her mind.

Well, the doctor had obviously said something to the nurses at the desk, since ey suddenly appeared in the labor room. By this time, Andrea was crying hysterically. meone arrived with a stretcher and they somehow managed to drag Mrs. Castaldo to it. By this time the lady was thrashing around and screaming, even though she emed to be still in a deep sleep. Now, this was a time when a few hospitals had just arted to allow some husbands to stay in labor rooms with their wives at the beginning their labors. This was one of those hospitals, and naturally there were a couple of sbands in the hall at that exact minute to witness the scene that followed.

Mrs. Castaldo's gown had been pulled off in the confusion. The glass I.V. bottle as on the floor, still attached by its tubing to Mrs. Castaldo's arm. Bump, bump, mp, it went along the floor, as the screaming naked lady with the blue head sticking t between her legs was raced to the delivery room. And at the end of the parade was ndrea, sobbing out loud and yelling, "I'm so sorry. I'm so sorry!"

Anyway, the doctor put on a pair of gloves and helped the rest of the baby into e world. Mrs. Castaldo probably didn't remember the circumstances of her eighth livery, since when she finally woke up a few hours later she seemed none the wiser. s for Andrea, she returned to sit with another patient in labor the very next day, and e staff wisely never assigned her to any patients of that particular obstetrician. She mained a total nervous wreck for the rest of her O.B. rotation, and insisted on necking between her patients' legs at least every two minutes.

On Andrea's last day of labor and delivery experience, she thought it was appening all over again. She ran out to the desk to get the nurses, screaming that she w the top of the baby's head.

It was a giant hemorrhoid.

It's safe to say that everyone was glad to see Andrea go. Most especially, ndrea herself.

Love Story

People said that they were the sweetest couple anyone had ever known. They
ıd met in college and it was love at first sight. Just like in the movies.

Alex and Helen got married during the summer between Alex's first and second
ar of medical school. They were young and had the whole world ahead of them. By
e time he graduated, they had a little boy. Two years after that, they had a girl. The
rfect family.

Just a few years after finishing his medical residency, Alex's practice was
ooming. When anybody asked for a referral for a good internist, Alex came to mind.
e was one of the favorites of all the nurses. Quiet and thoughtful, Alex was an
cellent practitioner and a kind and caring person. Everyone liked Alex.

Soon after, Helen began having stomach problems. Since she was a healthy
ung woman, nobody thought it could be anything serious. The absolute most she
uld have, they believed, was an ulcer. And even that wasn't likely.

Well, the G.I. series showed something worse. Helen had some kind of a mass
 the bottom of her stomach. She had further testing done, and everything pointed to a
iomyoma, a benign tumor arising from the smooth muscle. Helen would need surgery,
ıt she would be fine.

So the day of the surgery came, and everyone waited for the case to be over.
elen was to be brought to a private room in the step-down unit, and the nurses were
ally anxious to have Alex's waiting come to an end. He had been very nervous and
nse since he had learned of Helen's diagnosis, and they didn't like to see him like that.
emember, everyone knew and loved Alex.

They knew something was wrong as soon as they heard the recovery room
urse's voice. She was devastated. It seems the surgeon didn't like what he saw in the
perating room and had done a frozen section. The tumor was not benign. It was a
alignant leiomyosarcoma. And it had deeply infiltrated much of Helen's tissue.

Well, an hour or two later Helen was wheeled up from the recovery room with
lex at her side. The surgeon, who was one of their closest friends, was with them.
fter Helen was put to bed, they closed the door. None of the nurses was in the room,
nd so nobody knew exactly what went on. The surgeon emerged about ten minutes
ter, his eyes red and swollen. Shaking his head, he said nothing to the nurses. He
ouldn't.

110

After a short while Gina entered the room. She heard Helen say, "Oh, Alex, I so scared." Alex, hugging her, answered through his tears, "I'm scared too, Helen. They both began to sob, and Gina turned and walked out.

That was the beginning of the end for Helen and Alex. Shortly after Helen beg her chemotherapy, Alex decided he could no longer continue on in private practice. H life had changed too drastically for him to try to keep going as before. His priority w to spend time with Helen, and he couldn't do that with the long days and hours I routinely put in.

Helen did not do well with her chemotherapy. The size of the residual tum mass did not shrink, and she was sick every day. Her prognosis, from the beginnin had been poor. Alex became a part time house doctor in another hospital so that I could take care of his sick wife and their children. Helen passed away several mont later, and with her died a love story that never had a chance to be complete.

Oscars

"The leeches are coming."

At first, some of the nurses thought it was some kind of a joke. But those who knew and those who kept up with their nursing journals knew it was for real. The leeches were really coming.

Now, in trauma centers and big surgical units, leech therapy is not such a big deal. Routinely used in many postoperative replantation cases, leeches help in decreasing venous congestion. After surgical reattachment of a body part which has been traumatically amputated, there are times when the area swells up dangerously and compromises the blood supply to the site. And patients who have had body parts torn off or cut off nowadays are routinely sent to trauma units. So the trauma nurses are used to leech therapy.

But it's safe to say that the majority of nurses in America are not trauma specialists, and so the rest of us are not exactly used to working with worms. Anyway, here's how and why leeches are used. Sometimes, there is a problem postoperatively. The arterial blood gets in, but swelling keeps the venous blood from draining out. As one surgeon described it, it can be compared to the Lincoln Tunnel at rush hour where lots of lanes of traffic are merging to get into one of the tubes. As the cars dam up and can't flow smoothly, so does the blood as it's trying to drain back into the general circulation. There needs to be a way to get things flowing. In the tunnel, an extra lane or another tube under the Hudson River needs to be opened or the traffic will just about come to a stop. And with an arm or a finger or an ear, a method has to be established to get the blood moving out, or the newly re-attached part will suffocate and die.

Enter the leeches.

Leech therapy has been around for 2,500 years or so. Today's medicinal leeches come from special "leech farms" and are bred solely for use in reconstructive and cosmetic surgery. They are considered animals. Leech saliva contains a substance which acts as an anticoagulant, a vasodilator, and an anesthetic. So, in a nutshell, it painlessly promotes bleeding and drainage of the compressed area.

However, these darling little animals are real live brown worms. And they look and act like real live brown worms, who love to drink blood. People's blood. And guess how these wiggly worms are brought to the area where they are needed? By the nurses, of course.

Well, on this particular day in this particular hospital, a patient was havi[ng] trouble with his newly replanted finger. Having been torn off in an industrial accident, [it] had been reattached the day before. Now it was getting bluish and had all the signs [of] venous congestion. The nurses were applying local anticoagulation therapy by poki[ng] the area with a sterile needle and then squirting heparin on it. But that finger need[ed] something else. It was a classic case for leeches.

So the little guys arrived by Federal Express directly from the medicinal lee[ch] farm. They were delivered to the main pharmacy. The director of the pharma[cy] brought them up to the I.C.U. The leeches were in a regular fish tank, filled half wa[y] with water and covered on top with a cloth. Remember, leeches are worms and worm[s] like to crawl around, so there needed to be a barrier on the top of the tank. It would[n't] exactly be terrific to have worms crawling around the unit, everyone agreed.

The fish tank was put into the medication room refrigerator. Mary, the hea[d] nurse, put a sign on the refrigerator that read, "Open slowly and stay calm - leech[es] inside." Imagine what would happen if an unsuspecting nurse opened the door to gra[b] some insulin and found a glass tank filled with creepy crawly brown worms!

Everyone was great. The plastic surgeon took all the nursing staff into the repo[rt] room and explained how leech therapy works and what the nurses had to do. Then th[e] doctor went into the patient's room and explained everything to him. Remarkably, th[e] patient was very agreeable, although it probably was because he was somewh[at] sedated.

Wearing a glove, the doctor reached into the tank and took out the first leech. O[f] course the tank wasn't brought into the room, since that might have been a litt[le] overwhelming for the patient. The doctor held the leech over the bloody swollen sutur[e] line, and the leech started to go crazy. It obviously smelled the blood. Then th[e] flopping frenzied worm clamped its mouth right down on the finger and curled itse[lf] around it. Thankfully, the patient kept his eyes closed.

Well, that worm stayed put and seemed to begin to grow, right there befor[e] everyone's eyes. The literature said it would become engorged and satisfied with bloo[d] after about thirty minutes to an hour, but this guy was finished sucking within fiftee[n] minutes. By the time he was full, it looked like a small snake instead of a worm, and [he] let go and dropped to the floor. And then it started to crawl out of the room, leaving [a] bloody trail as he squirmed along.

Well, to say that was some sight is probably a bit of an understatement. Two o[f] the nurses started to scream, "Get him, get him!" So Mary, who was deathly afraid o[f] creatures, wound up throwing a blue chux over the fat overstuffed worm, and picking [it] up. As she said later, she had no choice. Everyone was running around and yelling an[d] she was afraid the patient was going to wake up and freak out or the worm would craw[l] nto another patients room or something. Doing what she had been told to do, she somehow was able to stuff the worm into the big bottle of alcohol on the window sill, which killed it.

And that started the leech therapy in the I.C.U. Every four hours a new leech had to be applied. Needless to say, there were a few nurses who just couldn't get involved, but that was O.K. JoAnn, one of the day shift nurses, loved those leeches and named them all "Oscar." The other nurses said she was nuts, but she liked to stick her gloved hand into the fish bowl and take her "Oscars" for a walk around the second floor, showing everyone her "pets."

Well. after two days of this, the finger began to improve. Along with the heparin therapy, the little worms were doing their jobs well. The last leech was applied five days after the surgery, and whatever Oscars were left in the tank were returned to the pharmacy.

A week or so later the patient, complete with a healthy finger, was discharged. The plastic surgeon wrote a letter to the hospital administration commending the nurses for their professionalism and support of this somewhat unorthodox procedure. It was an experience nobody would have wanted to miss.

Well, almost nobody.

A Head Nurse's Guide to Calling In Sick

xcuse	Response
Cramps	Come on. If all the females in the United States called in sick every month, the American work force would collapse. Take some Motrin and come to work.
Diarrhea	We have toilets at work. Get dressed and come in.
Sore Throat	Do you have drippy white blotches on your tonsils, big swollen glands, and a high fever? No? Then drink some orange juice, suck on some hard candy, and come to work.
Headache	Take 2 Tylenol and stand under a hot shower. By the time you get to work, your headache will be gone.
Cold	There are tissues in the clean utility room. We'll give you a box. And don't tell me you'll spread germs. Come on. This is a hospital. Do you think your few extra germs will make any difference?
Toothache	Call your dentist and make an appointment for before or after work. Then take 2 Tylenol and come in. You'll be too busy to think about your tooth.
Backache	Take a hot shower and come to work. Exercise is good for backaches.

Abdominal Pain	Can you describe it as a tearing agony which radiates to your back? No? Then you are not experiencing a dissecting aortic aneurysm. Come to work and the walking will make that gas move along.
Not Feeling Well	Give me a break. We don't all feel well every single day. You come to work. We'll give you a cup of coffee and you'll feel better. We need you here.
Morning Sickness	Come on. You have 7 months left in this pregnancy. Eat a cracker and come on in.
Flu	If you really have the flu, you'll be out for a week, not just today. These achy things are not real flu. Take a couple of tylenol and get in the car.
Calling in Sick On a Weekend or Holiday	You'd better bring in a note from your undertaker!!

Gone With the Wind

1. Mr. Williams had just finished his breakfast. "Ah, delicious," he announced to nobody in particular. Then, as he usually did after he ate, he removed his upper and lower dentures. Placing them carefully on his breakfast tray, Mr. Williams closed his eyes and fell asleep.

The dietary aide came by, put the cover on his tray, and took it back to the food truck. Mr. Williams' teeth, unfortunately, went with the tray.

Only the upper denture was found. The lower one either was thrown out or had melted away in the dishwasher.

2. Lynn loved to crochet. She made afghans and sweaters to give as gifts, and especially loved creating stuffed animals. It was Christmas time and Lynn had just finished a large crocheted turtle. Its shell was made of red and green granny squares, and everyone loved it. It sat up on display on top of the circular chart rack. One morning, however, the turtle disappeared. The nurses searched the unit, but it was gone. Somebody must have taken it, they reasoned, since obviously a big stuffed animal like that couldn't just get lost. Lynn was very upset. Her "baby" had been kidnapped.

The next day, Marlene confessed. She had thrown the turtle in a full laundry bag to "give it a bath" in the washing machine. Real funny. The laundry, naturally, had already been tossed down the laundry chute the evening before. Lynn raced down to the Laundry. As soon as she arrived, she saw her Christmas turtle sitting on top of one of the big washers. It had been rescued just before it hit the water and was being kept as a mascot by the Laundry department. Lynn grabbed the turtle and returned to the floor to kill Marlene.

3. Mrs. Patterson turned and tossed in her bed. She couldn't get comfortable. And to top it off, her hearing aid kept whistling. It was driving her crazy. So Mrs. Patterson took out her hearing aid and, to keep it safe, wrapped it up in a pile of tissues. She put it on the edge of her bedside stand and, after a short while, she fell asleep. The hearing aid, buried in the tissues, was scooped up by the housekeeper as she cleaned. It ended up in the trash.

It was never seen again. Nobody had any clue which of the forty million bags c garbage held the hearing aid. That was the end of it.

4. Mrs. Grayson came down to Radiology for a CT scan of her chest. As to many patients do, Mrs. Grayson had left the cardiac floor with her telemeter still aroun her neck and the leads in place. The Radiology nurse, realizing that the leads and wire would show up on the scan, took everything off Mrs. Grayson. She placed the monitc and whatever went with it on the sheet crumpled over the seat of Mrs. Grayson wheelchair.

At the end of the scan, someone else got Mrs. Grayson off the table. Noticin that the sheet was a bit soiled, she scooped it up and threw it in the dirty linen hamper This second person had no idea that Mrs. Grayson had come down with a telemeter And she certainly didn't leave the CT department with one.

When Mrs. Grayson was asked by her nurses where her telemeter was, she tol them she had no idea. Later that day, the Laundry supervisor called the Nursing Offic to say that they had found a strange looking portable radio. It had never gotten near washing machine. The telemeter was sent back up to the floor and the nurses though the whole thing was kind of funny. It really wasn't.

5. The narcotics were counted at the end of the day shift. At four o'clock, one c the evening nurses needed the keys. They were gone. The nurses searched the floc and checked everyone's pockets. No keys. They called the supervisor, who wasn exactly pleased to have to handle this problem, since she had just received three sic calls for the next shift. Two hours later, one of the day nurses called. She had foun the narcotic keys in her uniform pocket at home.

The keys were returned at the end of the evening shift by the day nurse's sor which most likely was against all hospital policies and probably some federal laws alsc But nobody said a word or made out any incident reports. Too much trouble.

6. Lorrie was in a mad rush. She had a million things to do when she left work. It was pay day, and she needed that money badly. So when the checks came up, sh took hers and placed it safely in what she thought was her pocketbook. When she wa getting ready to leave the hospital, she couldn't find the check. Lorrie realized that sh had accidentally put it in her friend Cathy's purse, one that looked very similar.

Lorrie went nuts when she couldn't reach Cathy. She couldn't get to the bank an never did her shopping. Cathy found the check late that night. Too bad.

7. Sue's patient died. After he was pronounced, Sue went into the room to d his post-mortem care. She wrapped the body in the shroud, and collected and labele

s clothes and belongings. Then everything went to the morgue. When her shift was ver, Sue went to put on her red sweater. But where was it? She remembered taking it ff when she started to wrap up the body. Uh, oh. Sue knew where that red sweater as. She had put it in the morgue bag with the her dead patient's clothing.

The body was long gone, along with the personal belongings. Everything was in e funeral home. So did she just forget about the sweater? Nope. Not Sue. She opped by that funeral home to retrieve it. After all, it was her favorite sweater. The ndertaker probably thought she was a bit nuts.

The Talking Clock

Everyone in the building was afraid it was going to happen one of these days. After all, Mrs. Wilkinson was getting old and she wasn't in very good health.

Mrs. Wilkinson's son, Richard, was totally dependent upon her. Although thirty-five, he had the mentality of a ten year old, and needed his mother for almost everything. There was no other family, and when Mrs. Wilkinson had her stroke, Richard was left alone. Except for the animals. Richard and his mother had three dogs and two cats, and the animals were Richard's friends. His only friends.

Mrs. Wilkinson was brought to the hospital, completely unconscious and extremely filthy. None of the neighbors had ever been inside their apartment before until Richard had run out to get help for his mother. It reeked. So now Richard was all alone. The neighbors, who always thought of them as quiet and peaceful people, sent food over for Richard and his pets, since it was obvious that he couldn't shop and cook for himself. They never went inside, though. It was too dirty.

And that's the way things went for a while. Richard walked the mile back and forth to the hospital every morning. He waited in the lobby until the security guard told him visiting hours were beginning, and then he walked upstairs to see his mom. Since Mrs. Wilkinson was in the step-down unit, the visiting hours ended for three hours and then started up again. During the break, Richard sat downstairs in the lobby. He watched television and colored in a big coloring book, which he carried to the hospital with him in the morning and then home again at night.

The Social Service department got involved with Richard right away. Arrangements were made for him to eat his meals at the hospital, and he was given help with all the paperwork involved with running his house. So Richard was doing O.K.

There was only one major problem. It was obvious that Mrs. Wilkinson was not going to get better. She was going to die. She had never been to any kind of a doctor, and it turned out that Mrs. Wilkinson had diabetes, heart disease, and high blood pressure. And that was just the basics.

She suffered from severe vascular disease, and when she was admitted, the toes of both feet were already becoming gangrenous from lack of blood supply. Two toes, in fact, looked quite a bit like pieces of dried up charcoal which were on the verge of simply snapping off in the bed.

The doctors and nurses sat with Richard on numerous occasions and told hi
just how sick his mother was. They told him that it looked very much as if she was n
going to come home from the hospital. Ever. But Richard just smiled and said that h
mother was going to get better. She would wake up any minute, he was sure. And h
talking clock was going to help her wake up.

It seems that Richard's prize possession, along with that big coloring book, wa
his talking clock. It worked on batteries, and when a button was pushed it began to pla
music. Then a loud voice announced, "The time is such and such. Time to wake up!
And Richard held that clock over his mother's head for hours on end, as it told h
mother to wake up. Over and over again. Whenever Richard put the clock down, h
took his mother's head in both his hands, and, rotating the head side to side, he calle
out at the top of his lungs, "Wake up, Sneaky Pete!" He did that continuously. Th
clock and the head. The clock and the head. The nurses told Richard not to turn h
mother's head so much, but he was really very gentle with her. He loved her a lot.

Now this went on for quite a while, and it quickly became apparent that Mr
Wilkinson was not going to die very soon. Her vital signs and heart rhythm were stab
as a rock. And Richard kept up the routine. He arrived early at the hospital lobby earl
in the morning and then went directly to the cafeteria for his breakfast. He then sat i
the same chair in the corner of the lobby and colored in his coloring book until it wa
time to visit. Then it was the talking clock and the "Sneaky Pete" chant until h
returned to the lobby. Then off Richard went to the cafeteria for lunch, and the da
progressed until it was time to go home and feed the dogs.

Richard never wore socks and this all took place in the dead of winter. And h
walked to and from the hospital in the same pair of brown beat up shoes. Nothin
anyone said could convince Richard to wear socks, even though it was obvious that h
feet were absolutely freezing. He just didn't like socks, he said.

One day, there was a small incident in the hospital lobby. It seemed a little bo
who was sitting with his mother wandered over to see Richard's coloring book. He to
his mother that the man in the corner was coloring pictures of naked ladies. And of a
things, he certainly was. It turned out that Richard's coloring book, which nobody eve
really glanced at before, was totally pornographic. Actually, it was quite gross. Whe
asked, Richard told the security guard that a man in his building had given it to him.
Richard seemed to be totally surprised that it had offended anyone. The decision wa
made to leave the coloring book in Mrs. Wilkinson's bedside stand, so if he wanted t
do so, Richard could color while he was alone in his mother's room. But not in a publi
place like the hospital lobby. Although Richard didn't really understand what th
problem was, he was his usual agreeable self.

At night, after Richard went home, the medical residents poured through the book, and their laughter and remarks echoed through the unit. It was as if sneaky little boys had found a dirty book. Real funny.

One day, Mrs. Wilkinson's crispy crunchy toe fell off in the bed. It just snapped off while she was being turned and the nurses threw it in the garbage. It really didn't seem like a body part; it was more like a piece of burned toast. Nobody told Richard.

After two months of care, Mrs. Wilkinson finally died. It really was sad, since it was kind of hard for Richard to grasp the idea that his mother would not ever be coming home. The hospital Social Service department and all the chaplains were terrific. They took care of everything and arranged for Richard to be looked after at home. After a few weeks, one of the chaplains and a social worker went to the apartment to see how things were going. They found that Richard had been sleeping in the bathtub so that his five animals could have the two beds. And the place was filthy. It was sad.

Many years have passed. Richard still lives in the apartment and he manages fairly well to take care of himself. He is a regular clinic patient and remains friendly to everyone. The clinic nurses call him regularly to see how he's doing and he is constantly reminded to bathe and wash his clothes. He looks like a mountain man, with his long bushy hair and beard. Richard carries the talking clock with him wherever he goes. He said he was mad at the clock at first, because it didn't wake up his mother. But after a while Richard realized that it wasn't the clock's fault. At least that's what he told everyone.

So life goes on for Richard. He manages. And he still never wears socks.

Danger

1. Donald Simmons was dying. He was a 32 year old intravenous drug abuser who had been sick with A.I.D.S. for the past two years. He now was hospitalized with P.C.P. pneumonia, common to patients with compromised immune systems. On top of that, he had developed a brain infection and active tuberculosis, all end stage manifestations of this horrible disease. He was semi-conscious and on a ventilator. Donald had what seemed like a thousand tubes and lines and was receiving multiple antibiotics and medications in a last ditch effort to try to prolong his life.

Donald also had no veins left from which to draw his blood, and the lab people had given up. So, as per protocol, the first year medical resident on the service was called to draw the blood from a vein in his groin.

Dr. Alan Crane was out of medical school a whole two months. He was a very hard worker, enthusiastic, and very well liked by the nursing staff. Anyway, Dr. Crane had a hard time getting the blood. Donald was restless and kept shifting himself around in the bed, unable to understand what the doctor was doing. Finally, the blood was drawn up into the syringe. Dr. Crane, using one hand to try to hold pressure on the site where the blood was drawn, attempted to squirt the blood from the syringe into the test tube with the other hand. Instead of pushing the needle through the top of the rubber stopper and injecting the blood into the tube, he jammed the bloody needle into his own hand.

2. Ellen Carter was also an I.V. drug abuser. She, like Donald, was in the I.C.U., terminally sick with A.I.D.S. One of her I.V. lines needed to be restarted that morning, and so her nurse, Catherine, went in to check her veins. To be on the safe side, Catherine asked Maureen to come and help her hold Ellen's arm still so as to prevent Ellen from moving her arm and pulling out the I.V. after the needle was inserted.

Catherine located a fairly good vein and Maureen held Ellen's arm steady as Catherine put the needle in. She then threaded in the plastic catheter and withdrew the needle. At that exact second, Ellen Carter jerked her arm sideways and Catherine, who was just putting the needle down, stuck that needle right into Maureen's finger.

123

3. Ken Adams also was a young man with A.I.D.S. Ken was critically ill, ar on a ventilator. His pneumonia was overwhelming, and it looked as if he wasn't goir to live more than a few days. Ken was practically comatose, but his cough refle remained very strong. Even with very frequent suctioning, copious amounts of mucu continuously gurgled in his endotracheal tube as he breathed.

Rita had just finished suctioning Ken, and was just about to reconnect th respirator tubing to the blue adaptor of Ken's airway. Suddenly he coughed violentl and a tremendous glob of yellow-green infected mucus shot directly into Rita's left eye.

4. Robert Jeffries had just died of A.I.D.S. His body had been tagged with a infectious disease sticker and sent to the morgue. Jane, who had been his nurse tha day, was cleaning up his room. She was in the utility room, scrubbing out the glas suction bottle which had recently contained Mr. Jeffries' infected mucus. The bottl slipped out of Jane's hand and smashed to the floor. A large piece of the broken glas bounced up and sliced Jane's hand.

All four of these health care workers were scared to death. They had thei baseline blood work drawn for H.I.V., as well as for hepatitis. And then they waited fo the results. As they had guessed, their baseline values were negative. Every month fo a full year after their exposures to the A.I.D.S. virus, they were retested. And they remained scared to death. All four of them did not convert. After the year was over Alan, Maureen, Rita, and Jane began to relax.

The H.I.V. virus is very fragile. It is not easy to catch A.I.D.S. And over the past few years there have been more and more safety measures developed to limi exposure. Sharps boxes are kept in every room, by every patient's bed. Needles shoulc go directly from the person's hand into the box. Also there are adapters without needles which limit ways that personnel can be stuck. Even the closed suction systems or ventilators prevent mucus from shooting into the air. And more and equipment is disposable, to reduce the risk while cleaning and caring for it.

But the danger remains.

Be very careful.

Burns

A lot of years had passed before she would let herself think about him. She must have pushed all those memories to the back of her mind, and even now her stomach still churns each time she begins to relive those days.

Elaine was a very young nurse, back then. She was, in fact no older than the patient who she tried so hard to forget. This was before there were burn centers and around the time that intensive care nursing was just beginning.

His name was Louie. She'll never forget the first time she saw him. Or rather saw what they did to him. Louie was coming home from the beach on a hot July day. He was driving alone on the highway, dressed just in a bathing suit. He was wearing beach sandals. There had been a terrible accident and some people were trapped in their car, which was beginning to smolder. Louie had pulled over to the side, jumped from his car and was attempting to pull the people out. And that's when the car exploded.

The people in the car were killed instantly, and Louie became a human torch. By the time Louie's flames were extinguished, he had sustained second and third degree burns over ninety-eight percent of his body. The only parts spared were the soles of his feet, where the sandals had been.

Elaine was working at a large county hospital. She was an evening nurse in the recovery room, and in those days they simply kept all the major cases overnight and called it an intensive care unit. So that's where Louie was brought. To a corner cubby in the recovery room.

Elaine had never seen Louie in the emergency room and to this day she remains grateful for that. But she'll never forget the exact moment she did see him for the first time. He had been rolled in to the unit and was on a Circle-Electric bed. His entire body was wrapped as if he were a mummy. The only openings in the dressings were small slits for his eyes and mouth. She noticed that his eyes had already swollen shut, so he probably couldn't see anyway. He breathed through a tracheostomy.

One of the things she remembers about burn care back then was the fact that they rarely sedated the patients. It would drop their blood pressure, the nurses were told. Even today, with all the high tech and drugs which patients are given, burn care hurts. Louie had nothing for pain. The doctors said that because most of his burns were deep

third degree, he shouldn't feel much pain anyway. All his nerve endings had bee
burned away.

But Louie was in agony. Of that, Elaine was certain. Until the day she dies
Elaine will never forget the first time Louie's mother saw him. She started to scream
"Oh, my God, Louie! Oh, my God." And Louie, who wasn't supposed to be able t
talk because of the trach, somehow was able to make sounds through it and said, "I'r
cool, Mom. Don't worry. I'm cool." She'll always remember those words.

Every day on every shift, those burn dressings had to be peeled off. And the
new dressings had to be wrapped around every inch of Louie's body. After that, silve
nitrate solution was poured from bottles to keep all the dressings soaked. Everythin
turned gray. The floors, the walls where the silver nitrate splashed, the nurses' uniforms
and the nurses' hands - - everything was gray.

Except Louie. Louie turned green. He developed the dreaded pseudomona
infection, the same bug which is still around today. And he smelled sweet, like
pseudomonas smells. Infection, which is still what most burn patients die of, wa
rampant back then. Techniques used now were never dreamed of. Elaine remember
doing Louie's dressings without even wearing gloves, doing one part of his body at
time. The worst thing she remembers about Louie, however, was the fasciotomy the
did on the second day of the burn injury, when Louie's extremities began to swell.

Even today this procedure is sometimes done to slit the burned tissue so that th
blood supply is not compromised. But it is not done now the way it was done bac
then. They simply took a scalpel and cut Louie, right from his shoulders to his finger
and from his groins to his toes. No anesthesia, no pain meds, no nothing. Elaine
remembers him screaming, even with that tracheotomy. Somehow, even though he
shouldn't have been able to, he could still scream. The memory of that still makes her
sick.

Everyone knew Louie was going to die. Nobody lives with burns as massive as
his were. Maybe if Louie had been an old man, the agony would have ended after a day
or two. But Louie was only twenty-two years old, and his organs were young and
healthy. So Louie lived on, along with his infections and his pain. Elaine remembers
that his mother brought in Plus White toothpaste for the nurses to brush Louie's teeth. I
seemed so ironic. Plus White toothpaste, when his whole body was charcoal. Or
green. Pseudomonas green.

She doesn't remember any skin grafting. Maybe that's because there wasn't any
non-burned skin to graft, or maybe it's because they didn't do grafting in those days.
And there certainly wasn't anything like pigskin to cover the burn injuries. There was
nothing. No debriding, no whirlpool, no nothing. Just that damn silver nitrate. They
would pour bottled saline on the bloody wet kling dressings to loosen them as they

ulled them off. Then they rewrapped everything with the new kling and saturated everything with the silver nitrate. There was no other treatment.

They say burned patients are always cold, because they lose all their heat as well as their body fluids through their missing skin. Well, Elaine still has vivid memories of Louie shaking so much that they were afraid he would fall off his Circle-Electric bed. All they could do was pile blankets on top of the cold wet dressings.

After two and a half weeks of his torture, Louie finally died. And the way he died added to the horror of this story. Louie's seventeen year old brother went in to see him, came out to the nurses' station, and simply said, "My brother is dead." He didn't cry. He didn't scream. He had no emotion. He simply said, "My brother is dead." And then he turned and left the hospital. Louie had died alone in the corner cubby, and his little brother was the one to find him dead.

Elaine and another nurse went in to do his post-mortem care. Without the whoosh of the Bird Respirator, the room was very still. They hardly spoke as they pulled all his dressings off. This was the first time they had seen his whole body at one time, since the dressings had always been done in pieces. As hard as she tried over the years to suppress the sight, she will never forget how Louie looked. His entire naked body was green and moist. His arms and legs looked like sticks. Green sticks with dried darker green crusts buried in the deep surgically made slits that ran the length of them. And he smelled sweet. So very sweet.

Elaine took care of several more horribly burned patients over the next few years. As bad and as horrifying as they were, nobody affected her more than Louie. When she finally left that hospital, a burn center was being built. To this day, Elaine believes firmly that each and every burn nurse is an angel sent from heaven. She also knows that the Louie's of that time are the reason that burn care has come so far today.

Rest in peace, Louie.

Peter the Peanut

He was so little when they first met him. At eighteen months old, he surely didn't belong in with all those adult patients. But things were different back then, and he truly needed the pulmonary I.C.U.

Peter had been sick for over a week, and had been getting progressively worse. They called it bronchiolitis, but whatever it was, it was bad. Peter couldn't breathe.

So before that first day had ended, Peter was intubated and placed on a ventilator. Besides the endotracheal tube, Peter had multiple I.V. lines, a foley catheter and a feeding tube. He looked like a little peanut, buried under a mound of equipment and lost in the big open adult I.C.U. And so Peter became known as Peter the Peanut.

Peter was the sweetest and most loving child the nurses had ever known. No matter what was done to him, he smiled around his E.T. tube and held out his arms to be picked up. This was a specialized pulmonary hospital and there were no other children in the whole building. A rocking chair was ordered especially so that Peter could be rocked. And was he ever rocked! It was very rare, indeed, to actually see Peter in his crib. Most of the time someone was sitting in that rocking chair with Peter on his or her lap.

Almost three months passed. Peter got better and was extubated five times, but five times he got sick again and had to be re-intubated. This was a long time ago, before multi-lumen catheters and arterial lines. So Peter had many cut-downs done and innumerable arterial sticks for blood gases. Peter's A.B.G.'s were gotten from his brachial arteries, and he got to know when the nurses were getting ready to stick him for blood. He cried soundlessly around his endotracheal tube when he saw the equipment coming, but he held out his little arms. And he knew that the sound of the suction machine meant he was going to be suctioned.

Peter the Peanut had more than his share of problems. He developed a stress ulcer, probably from the massive doses of steroids. He became septic. He had foot drop from one of the many intramuscular injections that he regularly received. He had sores in his mouth from the tube. And so on.

All through it, Peter remained the same lovable little peanut. Instead of pulling away from the nurses when they came near him, he continued to reach out to them and smile. He loved it when the nurses rocked him and sang to him. His mom shared him with the nursing staff, and Peter became everyone's baby.

128

Now, remember that this was before the time of CT scans, so the only picture they had of Peter's lungs were routine chest x-rays. And they continued to show the same types of inflammatory patterns. Today maybe someone would think that this baby had PCP pneumonia, but there was no such thing as AIDS back then. So the plan was to keep trying to reduce that inflammatory disease with medications and antibiotics. That's all they could do.

Well, after those three months had passed, it was decided it was time to bronc Peter and take a look down into the lungs. The doctors hadn't done this before since they would have had to give Peter general anesthesia, and they were certain this would make things much worse. But now, they were running out of time.

So early one morning, Peter the Peanut was taken off to the operating room. His mom and his nurses went with him so he wouldn't be with strangers. After all, the nursing staff was now very much considered Peter's family. Peter went in and everyone just waited for word as to what the doctors would find.

When the answer came, it was unbelievable. There was a peanut tucked down in Peter's right lung. A big peanut, which never showed up on any of his x-rays. The doctors retrieved it through their bronchoscope, and that was that!

Peter's mother remembered that the night before he got sick, he had been playing with his seven year old sister. They were eating Crackerjacks. So Peter must have aspirated a peanut, and nobody knew it.

Well, without that peanut hiding down in Peter the Peanut's lung, he started to get better fast. Within a few days he was extubated and eating and running around the I.C.U. with his I.V. pole. Peter the Peanut was now a normal happy toddler, who obviously had forgotten how sick he had been. He certainly was ready to be transferred back to the pediatric ward in the general hospital, but his I.C.U. nurses wouldn't hear of that.

Instead, Peter the Peanut was moved to the little step-down isolation room right off the unit and kept there until he was ready to go home. The day before discharge they had a big party for Peter the Peanut. Every staff member bought Peter toys and clothes, and there were balloons and streamers everywhere. Peter zoomed up and down the halls and in and around that pulmonary I.C.U. in his new big blue plastic car with the smiling face painted on the front. He was so happy, but not as happy as his nurses!

Peter's mom used to come to the hospital every day by subway, but that wasn't the way they went home. They left in a stretch limousine, packed with all his presents. And right there in the middle of all the toys was Peter the Peanut, smiling and waving goodbye to the nurses who loved him so much.

129

Confused Patients Can - And Do

1. - - - Chew on their I.V. tubings until they actually gnaw a hole through them and the liquid runs into the bed.

2. - - - Finger paint the side rails with the contents of their diapers.

3. - - - Manage to climb up and over their side rails and then fall right on the floor.

4. - - - Squirm down in their wheelchairs until they are strangling on their poseys.

5. - - - Pull their top sheets completely off by using just the first two fingers of their restrained hands.

6. - - - Tip over their I.V. poles by pulling steadily and firmly on the I.V. tubing.

7. - - - Horde a mouthful of pills under their tongues and spit them all over the bed two hours later.

8. - - - Drink from their urinals and pee in their water pitchers.

Bill

She talked about him once in a while, not all that much. After all, Helene was a
private type of person. But everyone knew how she felt about him.

Both Helene and Bill were divorced, and she had met him at her son's softball
game. It was sort of like fate had stepped in, two single parents watching their sons
play ball. You know.

They hadn't started dating yet; it was more of a "thing" than a relationship. But
they both knew it was coming. They had so much in common and they just enjoyed
being together. They had fun.

Helene seemed upset one morning. Bill had gotten sick over the weekend, she
said, and he had been admitted to the hospital. Something abdominal, she said.
Probably an intestinal problem. He had been vomiting and had severe abdominal pains.
Helene, being an x-ray technologist, thought it could have been any number of things.
He could have some kind of inflammatory process like diverticulitis or even Crohn's
disease, or possibly an intestinal obstruction. Her mind ran through all of the
possibilities, some much worse than others.

Well, an hour or so later Helene came to get Marge. She was having problems
with an I.V. Somehow the tubing had gotten tangled up in knots and it was hooked
through and around the sleeve of her patient's gown. And the nasogastric tube had
dripped all over the gown, and now it needed to be changed. No problem, Marge told
Helene, as they walked slowly down the hall to X-ray room six. Helene started to talk
about Bill and how sick he was. She really seemed upset. It dawned on Marge that Bill
must be the patient in X-ray room six, the one with the spaghetti tangle of I.V. tubing.
Oh, my, thought Marge. It must be a little strange to take x-rays of a guy who's almost
your boyfriend.

Just before they reached room six, Helene got called to the phone. Marge
walked into the room by herself and found the patient sitting on the edge of a chair. He
greeted her with a big hello, and Marge thought to herself that this man was really
friendly. The I.V. tubing was tied in a knot right through the sleeve, just the way it gets
when somebody tries to stuff the I.V. bag in the wrong way. Then Marge looked at the
man's face and stopped short. He must have been seventy-five years old.

Marge looked at the patient's name band. Yep, she said to herself. That's him
alright. His name was William something or other. Bill. Her face was beet red by this

time. Marge helped the man stand up so she could untangle him from the I.V. He mu
have been six inches shorter than she was and Helene was even taller than Marge. A
when Marge finally got the gown off, she realized that Bill had a colostomy sitting rig
there on his distended abdomen.

"Uh, duh," stammered Marge. "So you're a friend of Helene." The man smile
"Oh, yes," he answered. "Isn't Helene a lovely girl? I'm really a lucky guy to have m
up with her!" Marge hesitated. "Heh, heh," she mumbled, unable to think of anythi
lucid to say to him. After a few minutes the patient, Bill, was tied into his clean and d
x-ray gown. Marge helped him climb up onto the high table to wait for Helene. S
covered him with a blanket. "Oh, you are an angel," teased Bill. I'm a lucky guy
have both of you."

Not knowing what to say, Marge just patted Bill's hand and left the room. S
tried to pull herself together. This was the Bill who Helene was falling in love with
Oh, not that there was anything wrong with him, but to be perfectly honest, she cou
not imagine why a beautiful thirty year old blond would be attracted to a short dum
old man with a colostomy. Maybe, though, Marge suddenly thought, Helene did
know he had the colostomy. That's it, she was suddenly sure. How could Helene ha
any idea? They were just getting to know each other. Oh, my God, Marge said
herself. If Helene walks into that room and sees that big distended belly with i
glistening colostomy stoma, she'll be so shocked that she'll faint. I have to break this
her gently.

Well, Marge began to run down the hall in order to head off Helene before s
walked into X-ray room six and discovered the guy she loved lying on the table with h
colostomy bag in full view. It was her duty to protect their fragile new love. And the
suddenly she saw Helene. Helene had come through the back corridor and was ju
about to enter X-ray room six.

"Helene, stop!" screamed Marge. "There's something I have to tell you." Hele
looked puzzled. "What's wrong?" she asked. Marge took Helene by the hand a
pulled her down the hall to the window. "Listen, Helene," said Marge, trying to be
gentle and understanding as possible. "I just met your Bill. He's so very different fro
how I pictured him, but if you love him that's all that counts. He seems like a ve
sweet man. But I don't think Bill ever told you that he has a colostomy, and he real
seems to be obstructed. I really feel it's my duty to tell you that he may be a very si
man. I don't want you to walk into the room unprepared, so I wanted you to know wh
to expect. If, I mean, when Bill gets out of the hospital, you will be able to cope bett
with what lies ahead."

Helene just stared at Marge. "Are you, by any chance, trying to tell me that yo
think the little man in X-ray room six is the Bill I met at the softball game and the guy

ve a crush on?" she asked slowly. Marge hesitated. "Well, isn't he? You told me
at was him. And his name is Bill."

"Oh, my God," laughed Helene, shaking her head. "Marge, you are totally
sane. You are a crazy person." The man in room six is a great grandfather. I just
iished speaking to his wife out in the waiting room. My Bill is thirty-one years old,
d in another hospital, with what I just found out turned out to be a kidney stone."

After a few minutes, Marge and Helene walked into X-ray room six together.
)h, here are my two girlfriends," called out the patient, Bill something or other. You
ls remind me of my granddaughters. They're just as sweet as you are, and they just
ve to tell jokes. Do you like to tell jokes?"

Helene looked at Marge. "Well, well, well," she said to Bill. "Do I have a
nny story to tell you!"

The Hypochondriacal Nurses Association

One evening, as Becky was looking in the Merck Manual for a disease she knew he was getting, it hit her just how many times she had done that during the past year. Maybe she was becoming just a bit neurotic, she thought, laughing as she skimmed through the pages.

Becky thought back to when she was a student nurse, a lifetime ago. In those days, she and most of her classmates worried that they had symptoms of lots of exotic illnesses. In fact, as they learned about them, they realized how possible (or probable) it was that they had them. She particularly remembered the afternoon when she told her roommate that she was pretty certain that she had Yellow Fever. Right there in New York City, she had contracted Yellow Fever. Yeah, O.K.

But that was when they were kids, when diseases were new to them. It was different now. She was a nurse with a hundred years of experience. She should be a little wiser now. Sure.

The diseases Becky worried about now were different. She knew she wasn't likely to contract malaria or typhoid fever, but the routine stuff was very real to her. Not only real, but almost certain. After all, look at everything she saw day in and day out. Why should she be spared? She was due to get at least one horrible illness, wasn't she?

When Becky got a headache, it was a brain tumor. If she had body aches or fever with the headache, it was not the flu or something like that. No, it was meningitis. And if the headache came on suddenly, the only thing it could possibly be was a leaking cerebral aneurysm. No doubt. A fever with swollen glands meant AIDS. If she was constipated, she had an obstructing colon cancer. Low back pain never was muscular; it was renal colic. And she just knew she would never pass that kidney stone that she definitely had; she needed to have stents and all kinds of fancy things done. Upper back pain was worse, certainly. People don't get that too often, so when she had it, it was a symptom of a dissecting aortic aneurysm. No doubt.

When Becky felt tired, that was the beginning of leukemia. And even more certainly if she had a bruise or two anywhere. And lower abdominal distress or bloating had to mean ovarian cancer. She would have welcomed a simple ruptured appendix, but that would be too easy to treat. It had to be ovarian cancer. A swollen gland in her neck meant Hodgekins Disease or another lymphoma; mono would be too simple. She would spontaneously recover from mono.

134

A pain in the side of her chest meant pulmonary emboli. Becky remembered tl day at work, not too long ago, when she was certain that she had a spontaneo pneumothorax, in spite of the fact that she had eaten an entire bag of Doritos for lunch That time she was cured by a good burp. Just in time to avoid the chest tube.

Her friend Marilyn was once very certain she had tuberculosis. She went dow and had a chest x-ray and everything. She had a cold. It turned out the night sweats sl worried so much about came from going to sleep every night with her electric blank turned up to "Cook." Hmmnn.

Carol was positive she had pericarditis. Could that stretching and reaching sl did with her new exercise tape have anything at all to do with her sore chest? Naahh Of course not. And Connie knew she had bone cancer in her foot. It turned out to t some kind of boo boo that went away. Tincture of time took care of that one.

And this flesh eating bacteria thing that was hitting the newspapers and the T.\ news. Oh, lots of nurses had that. Any little scratch that stayed red meant that the fles eating bacteria was about to spread and destroy their bodies.

Judy was really worried. Every time she washed her hair in the shower, sh tasted soap. She must have had some type of fistula or communication somewhere The soap went right through and onto her tongue. Could it just have dripped into he mouth? Of course not.

One of the more fancy illnesses was self-diagnosed by Peter. His allergies ha become impossible. His eyes and nose constantly dripped. Peter checked his book and decided he had a histamine secreting tumor. He was very very worried about tha one.

Last month John had a toothache. He had to get to the dentist before th infection around the tooth (which he absolutely knew existed) spread through hi bloodstream to his brain and caused a brain abscess. And Susan had a slight postnasa drip, which most people would blame for the cause of her occasional cough. But nc Susan. She knew the real reason. It was an inoperable lung tumor.

And so on.

People who say, "It's just a cold," or "It's just a pulled muscle," or "It's just som viral thing," are living in their dream worlds. The Hypochondriacal Nurses Associatio knows best. Its members know what's really going on. Now, please excuse Becky. She has pain in her lower abdomen and she has to check her textbooks to find out th latest treatment to repair her perforated bowel. Oh, no! It looks as if she will need temporary colostomy. Nothing less for the president of the Nurses Hypochondriaca Association.

Oh, well.

Cockroaches

The nurses had seen a couple of bugs once or twice before. They seemed to have crawled out from under the ice machine. But nobody thought much about that; after all even in hospitals there are insects. You can't really help it. Somehow they just get in.

Well, this particular day Julie was in room 437, giving Mrs. Lancaster a bath. Room 437 was the last room in the unit, right next door to the pantry where the nourishments were kept. Mrs. Lancaster slept a lot, and at this particular time, she was drowsy but awake.

Julie had just dipped the washcloth in the bath basin and was rinsing off the soap when she noticed the bug crawling on Mrs. Lancaster's pillow. At that exact moment, a second one marched right across the lady's cheek. Julie grabbed the wet washcloth and swatted Mrs. Lancaster across her face, trying to knock the bug off. Mrs. Lancaster's eyes opened wide, just in time to see bug number three scamper along the sheet.

The patient, in contrast to Julie, did not get excited. "Is that what I think it is?" she asked quietly. "Yes, yes, it's a bug!" screamed Julie. "A disgusting roach!" And Julie, ever so professionally, ran out of the room.

Well, after a bit of brilliant investigating, the nurses realized that the little creatures were coming right through the wall from the pantry next door. Mrs. Lancaster was moved out of that bed and out of that room to a different room down the hall. Julie, to nobody's surprise, did not help.

Room 437 was closed and the Environmental Services Department was notified. The exterminator arrived a short time later and announced that those bugs were baby cockroaches. He said he was reasonably confident that there was a nest underneath the ice machine in the pantry and that's where the roaches were coming from. At this point, each and every person was thinking about the last time they had gotten ice from that ice machine. Had they seen anything mixed in with the ice? Anything dark? They tried to remember.

How very disgusting, everyone said. Can you imagine having a cockroach nest in a hospital? No big deal, said the exterminator. You can find roaches anywhere. Hospital or not. He'd take care of it, he said. Not to worry.

So the pantry was considered off limits. Someone, not one of the nurses, cleaned out all the shelves, and then the exterminator did his thing. He sprayed or set off some

136

kind of a bug bomb or something. And he did the same thing in room 437. Nobod
really wanted to know exactly what he did. Then the pantry and room 437 were seale
off and yellow tape, just like the kind they use in crime scenes, was put around the are
It looked just a little obvious, like something was going on. When people asked wh
had happened, they were told that there was a leak, since it would have been a litt
awkward to say this med-surg floor was infested with cockroaches. Political
incorrect, as they say nowadays.

Well, the next morning it was time to open the doors and see what, if any, kind
results they had gotten.

Unbelievable.

The floor of the pantry was dark brown. It was covered with what looked like
thousand dead bugs. And they were not babies; most of them were big fat cockroache
It was absolutely gross. And there were about fifty bugs in room 437. Yuk!

One of the housekeeping people swept up the bugs. He wasn't really grossed ou
in fact he seemed to think it was kind of funny. The nurses didn't agree. They wante
to puke.

Well, after a repeat performance of spraying and/or bombing those rooms, the
were washed down and scrubbed and pronounced ready for use. The nursing sta
swore they would never again use that ice machine, but you know that promise wasr
kept. Nobody ever saw another bug, but to this day room 437 is known as th
"cockroach room." And the nurses still keep a lookout from the corners of their eye
when they are doing their nursing care in there.

Doctor Sturtz and His Dad

He looked like a bird. He really did. Always a little man, he was now shriveled
ꞏd emaciated. And without his false teeth, which no longer fit, he looked even more
ꞏthetic.

Mr. Sturtz was very sick. In fact, he was dying. Almost ninety years old, he
ꞏas tired of living that way and was ready to go. That's what he told everyone. "I'm
ꞏady to go," he said. And he said it all the time. "Leave me alone and let me go. I'm
ꞏady."

Mr. Sturtz had metastatic colon cancer. He got lots of pain medicine, though,
ꞏd most of the time he was pretty comfortable. The drugs were doing a good job. He
ꞏally shouldn't have been in the hospital, either, most people said. Mr. Sturtz obviously
ꞏeded care, and lots of it, but he would have been fine in a skilled nursing home or at
ꞏme with Hospice care. However, in those days, there wasn't any Hospice, and
ꞏsides that, his son wouldn't have allowed it anyway. Mr. Sturtz's son was a doctor, a
ꞏmily doctor on the staff of that same hospital. And he wanted his father right there.

Dr. Sturtz spent a big part of his day with his father. Actually, he was a
ꞏonderful nurse to him. He bathed him and turned him and put lotion all over his
ꞏinny arms and legs. He did all of this even though he knew very well that the nurses
ꞏok good care of his father. It was just something he had to do. Mealtime was
ꞏmething else. It was obvious that Dr. Sturtz equated food with love, because his main
ꞏbjective was to see to it that his father ate. The poor little man had no appetite, but Dr.
ꞏturtz stood at that bedside three times a day, every day, and packed his mouth with
ꞏod. "No more," Mr. Sturtz would whimper. "No, Dad, you have to eat," prodded the
ꞏod doctor. "Open your mouth! You have to get your strength back!"

Julie and Carol were Dr. Sturtz' favorite nurses. It would be lovely to say that he
ꞏas one of their favorite doctors, but this was not exactly the truth. He was a very nice
ꞏan, but Dr. Sturtz should have retired years ago, they all thought. He just didn't know
ꞏnough any more, and it showed in his medical care.

This one particular night, Dr. Sturtz came in with two gifts. One was for Julie
ꞏnd one was for Carol. He gave them the presents, thanking them for all the T.L.C. they
ꞏad been giving his father. In the boxes were little packages of soap and perfumes.
ꞏlie And Carol were really flattered. They knew that Dr. Sturtz was a widower and

138

lived alone, and that he didn't have much extra time for shopping. Especially with the time he spent with his dad.

Thanking him profusely, the two nurses told Dr. Sturtz that they would take ext care of his dad that night, and that he should go home and go to bed early. They kne he'd call to check on his father just before the eleven o'clock news came on, though. H always did.

Well, it was close to eight o'clock and there wasn't too much going on that nig The floor was quiet and all the evening care had long been done. Julie walked down the end of the hall to check on Mr. Sturtz. He wasn't in his bed. Julie turned the lig on and looked around the room. There on the floor under the sink was Mr. Sturtz Naked as a jaybird, he was lying in a little puddle of blood, and was babbling out lou obviously totally confused.

Carol came flying down the hall when she heard Julie call her name. She ju knew something had happened. The two nurses easily lifted Mr. Sturtz back to be since he didn't weigh more than seventy or eighty pounds. As they did so, they sa where the blood was coming from. He had two gashes on his left arm, and another o on his penis.

"What are we going to tell Dr. Sturtz?" Carol and Julie said at the same tim staring wild eyed at each other. And then they just burst out laughing. The poor litt man didn't know they were laughing; he was kind of out of it by then. It really was funny, but then again, it sort of was.

Well, of course that was the one night that Dr. Sturtz called bright and early "I'm taking your advice," he said when they answered the phone. "I know that you gir take such good care of my dad that tonight I'm going to relax and turn in early. I kno he's in good hands with you."

"Umm, Dr. Sturtz," stuttered Julie. "I have something to tell you. You know th your father was acting a bit confused before, right? Well, it seems he forgot where was and climbed out of bed over the side rails. He kind of fell on the floor and sort cut himself." And then Julie held her breath and waited for the response.

Dr. Sturtz started to laugh. "Well, I guess there's some life in the old buzzar yet," he said. "See, I knew he wasn't anywhere near dying, like everyone seemed think!" Then he wished Julie a good night and hung up the phone, sounding happi than he had been in a long time.

It wasn't very hard for Carol and Julie to figure out why Dr. Sturtz was so elate The fact that his father had enough will and strength to climb out of bed meant that t old man still wasn't ready to die. The fall meant nothing to Dr. Sturtz. In his eyes, h father was stronger than ever.

139

For two days, everything was the same. The poor little man remained the way he
d been for the past week, sick as could be, but no worse. Then one evening, while
arol was in the medication room and Julie was on the phone in the nurses' station, Mr.
urtz died. Dr. Sturtz walked down the hall to see his dad, and apparently found him
ad. Dr. Sturtz pulled the oxygen catheter from his father's face, threw it across the
om, and screamed out loud, "My father is dead!" Then he strode out of the nurses'
ation.

From that day on, Dr. Sturtz never spoke one word to Julie or Carol. He
mpletely ignored them, except for glaring in their direction when he came within
enty feet of them. It was as if he blamed them for his father's death. Dr. Sturtz'
rsonality, in fact, totally changed towards all nurses. He seemed to have no use for
y of them and spoke, coldly and impersonally, only when it was absolutely necessary.
ver the years, Dr. Sturtz' practice has become very small and he is now semi-retired.
nd he still avoids nurses.

Alcohol

She took her first drink at the age of thirteen. By the time she started her senior year of high school she was, most probably, a practicing alcoholic.

Cheryl was a great person and was very easy to love. She was funny and she cared about everybody. She was a wonderful friend. Cheryl never got drunk in public. Not being a party girl, she liked to spend time at home. And that's where she drank.

Cheryl had gotten married at the age of twenty, and by the time she was twenty-four, she had two children. Cheryl's husband knew she had a drinking problem, and it wasn't long before there were serious problems in their marriage.

As the years passed, things got worse. She had blackouts and many lost weekends. Her drinking gradually began to affect her job. Never being drunk at work, there were, however, lots of times when she was really hung over. Her hands shook and she looked terrible. And her attendance got worse and worse.

Each time Cheryl got sick, she swore that she would never drink again. She tried to get help. She really wanted to stop. Cheryl went through detox and rehab many times. She went to A.A. meetings and counseling. She was very aware that her alcoholism could really kill her. She knew that she could never be cured of her disease, but that she could learn to keep it under control. She tried so hard. But it didn't work.

Cheryl was admitted to the intensive care unit of her community hospital many times. By this time, her marriage had broken up and her husband had custody of the kids. As sad as that was for Cheryl, she knew it was right. After all, if she couldn't even take care of herself, she knew she couldn't take care of her children. She developed cirrhosis of the liver and esophageal varices, and the varices began to break open and bleed. Once very pretty, her abdomen was now hugely distended with ascitic fluid. She came close to dying a few times, and each time that happened she prayed for another chance. Cheryl wanted to live. She loved her husband and wanted to be able to once again be a mother to her children.

But with each bleeding episode, things got worse. Cheryl became jaundiced and her once beautiful brown eyes were now surrounded by yellow. Her teeth were stained from blood which oozed from her swollen gums. With the big tubes in her nose and the I.V. lines in her neck, Cheryl now was a horrible sight.

Her husband couldn't stand to see her that way any more so he stopped coming to see her. He refused to bring the children either, believing that the sight of their mother might terrify them, and as he told the staff, he did not want them to remember their mother that way. And Cheryl's parents, who could not understand the overwhelming control that the alcohol had over their daughter, refused to see her again. Ever.

On her last admission to the I.C.U., Cheryl came in barely conscious. They called it alcoholic encephalopathy, which is known in most hospital lingo as "the pickled brain syndrome." By this time, her kidneys had become affected, and she was in renal failure. Cheryl's body was being poisoned by its own toxins and she was bleeding again.

As fast as they transfused Cheryl, the blood came pouring out of the tube which drained her stomach. Cheryl's failing liver could not secrete the factors to allow her blood to clot. So it kept pouring from the open varicose veins in the top of her stomach and her esophagus. The suction machine sucked that blood up and out through the tube into the big bottle on the wall. Soon everyone realized that they were wasting precious blood products.

And so Cheryl was allowed to die. She was alone, except for the nurses who took turns holding her hand and talking to her and telling her that it was O.K. and her fight was over. There was an intern, one of the nurses remembered, who just couldn't deal with this. He kept pacing around with tears in his eyes, saying over and over again "I just don't know what to do." He felt as if he had failed her, never before having been in the position of just stepping back and letting one of his patients die. He was too new, too young.

They watched and they waited. Even though it really didn't matter, the bed was up in Trendelenburg position as with any shocky patient. So the blood, which by this time was also coming out of Cheryl's rectum, flowed up toward her shoulders. It dripped down over the sides of the bed, making red puddles on the floor. They put bath towels down to catch the flow, and soon the plopping noises of the blood hitting the towels became very loud and sad. And so, as they watched, the life blood literally drained out of Cheryl, and then it was over.

Alcohol, the drug, had claimed another victim.

142

A Day In The Life Of A Hospital

1. The E.R. says they can't hold the patient any longer.

2. Mr. C. is lying on the floor.

3. Pharmacy says they never got the order even though they've been sending the drug for two days.

4. There's no more vented pump tubing and I have to hang my next T.P.N. bottle right this minute.

5. Mrs. P. went to X-ray in her bed and now she's back and her bed is all destroyed and you'll have to re-do it.

6. Nuclear Medicine says a nurse has to stay down there with the patient and the scan will take at least three hours.

7. Dr. B. needs a bed for his patient and doesn't want to hear about our bed problems.

8. C.C.U. is coming over with that patient right now.

9. Mr. L. just pulled out his cantor tube.

10. Two lumens of Mr. K's triple lumen catheter are clogged solid and he has no veins and needs to start on lidocaine right now.

11. Guess who pulled out her foley catheter again?

12. The PTT was never drawn and the last one was >150 and Dr. S. is having a giant fit.

13. Dr. E. is on the phone and wants to know all about Mrs. J. and I told him her nurse is at break and he's going crazy.

14. You'll have to move your quiet sweet little man in 228 up to telemetry and take a STAT admission -- an E.R. patient restrained in four point leathers who is in raging D.T.'s.

15. Mr. T. went into V. tach. and somehow the alarms were off and the monitor didn't catch it.

16. We need to start dopamine right now and there are no more IMED's.

17. Mr. P. got his morning insulin, but the tube feeding was on hold and now his blood sugar is 23 and he doesn't look so good and Dr. P. is having a fit.

18. There are no more N/G tubes and Mrs. T. is vomiting non-stop.

19. We are out of morphine and the pharmacy just closed.

20. A patient is being intubated on 6-West and we have no beds and no orders to transfer anyone and we have to take him right now.

21. Mrs. L. is in pulmonary edema and we have to start peritoneal dialysis right away.

22. Mr. P. just passed out on the commode and guess what? He is on absolute bedrest.

23. Mrs. G's bed is soaked again and this is the seventh time this shift and the resident won't let us put in a foley.

24. Mr. T. is incontinent of diarrhea in the recliner and the family is here and knows it and the orderly is at dinner and the patient is much too heavy to move and the family is going wild.

25. I think Mr. J. sort of just extubated himself.

26. Mr. K. just voided in his water pitcher.

27. Mr. G. climbed out of bed and pooped in the garbage pail in the corner of his room.

28. Mr. L. is NPO for endoscopy and he got his tray by mistake and ate everything and as soon as the doctor takes a look through the scope he is going to know and he's

going to kill us.

9. The O.R. is calling for the patient and there's no consent, no CBC, and no H & P.

0. Mrs. L. is walking out of the unit stark naked except for a posey vest and her pocketbook which is draped over her left arm.

1. C.S.R. has no more hypothermia blankets and Mr. T.'s temp is a hundred four point six.

2. It's the nursing office. I know you came in O.T. just to help us but they're pulling you to 5-East.

3. The chest drainage was never hooked to wall suction and the lung is not expanded and Dr. H. is screaming.

4. There's a naked patient standing in front of the desk.

Bill and Mama

She had raised him alone and they were always very close. In fact, most people said they were too close. A mama's boy, they called him. It wasn't normal.

Bill's health wasn't so good either. He had an inflammatory bowel disease, which, from time to time, made him sick. And his mother fussed over him and worried about him. Terribly. Always. Since he was a baby.

Bill was now twenty-eight years old and he lived at home with his mother. He had never held a real job. Each time he started to work, he quit. It was never right for him. The work was too boring. Or too hard. Or meaningless. Or too far to drive.

So Mama, who had lots of money, supported Bill. She told him he really didn't have to go to work. Mama and Bill were very close. He never had a real friend, never really needed one. He had Mama.

One day Bill really got sick. His bowel became very inflamed and he was admitted to the hospital with all the signs of an acute abdomen. Tests showed a perforated colon and Bill ended up with major surgery and a colostomy. His postoperative course was anything but simple. There were several trips back to the operating room, and before a month had passed, Bill ended up with a couple of draining wounds and fistulas. He sported four ostomy bags on his abdomen, one for the colostomy and three to catch the draining pus before it ate up his skin. He was a mess.

It was almost impossible to get Mama away from Bill's bedside. She hovered and fussed over him constantly. She bathed him and powdered him and fluffed his pillows. She tucked his blankets in just the way he liked them. And Bill seemed to love it. Why shouldn't he? He never knew any other way.

Well, Bill became very attached to one particular nurse. Nancy took care of him five evening a week, and she was wonderful with him. While most of the other nurses couldn't help resenting Bill's mother and making remarks about their relationship, Nancy didn't. From the start she accepted her and the major role she played in Bill's life. And Mama seemed to like Nancy a lot. Nancy was Mama's link to the hospital system. Nancy was Mama's special nurse, which surprised everyone since they really thought Mama wanted Bill all to herself.

Before long, the other nurses began to tease Nancy. They told her they thought Bill was falling in love with her, and they kidded her that she probably was his first

146

girlfriend. Nancy just laughed and told them they were being silly. She was just hi
favorite nurse.

Bill really was sick. It was a long time before he could eat or be weaned off hi
many antibiotics. He needed pain medicine around the clock. He lost weight and wa
very weak. And Nancy was there for him the entire time. Mama and Bill simpl
tolerated the other nurses. They were just there to fill in for Nancy when she was of
duty.

Finally, the doctors started making plans for his discharge. And one fine night
with his mother right there at the bedside, Bill asked Nancy to marry him and move int
the house with him and Mama. Nancy, who never saw it coming, let Bill down a
gently as she could. But things in that room were never the same again. Bill jus
wanted to go home, and he refused to speak to Nancy. Mama behaved in the same way
and it was obvious that Nancy had rejected THEM, not just Bill. It really was time t
go home.

Well, Mama made all the arrangements. This was before the days of discharg
planning and things like that. But even if help had been available, it was doubtful tha
Mama would have been interested. It was Mama's show to run. She decided that Bil
was going to move into her bedroom, into her double bed, in fact. There was plenty o
room for the two of them in that big bed, she said. She ordered a bunch of Chux an
urine bottles and bedpans, and she was going to nurse her son back to health. All by
herself. She knew now, she said, that there was not meant to be anyone in their live
but them. And Bill agreed.

So Bill and Mama left the hospital together. There were no real hard feelings
just a sense of disappointed acceptance on their parts. The nurses just shook thei
heads.

Was this a weird situation? Sure. Was there any funny stuff going on at home
like some people insinuated? Most likely, not. It's a big world and it takes all kinds o
people to live in it.

There are probably lots of Bills and Mamas out there. And they do just fine.

Just Pickin'

Marilou remembered Carol Brownley very well. Just ten days earlier she had taken care of her in the Radiology department. Carol had been in renal colic, and had been in agony. Patients who go through renal colic liken it to giving birth. It hurts!

Even with the morphine, Carol had experienced terrible kidney spasms, and had vomited almost continuously during the intravenous pyelogram. And the films showed quite a large kidney stone. No wonder it hurt, thought Marilou.

Well, during an average day, Radiology nurses see an awful lot of patients. To be honest, most of them are forgotten after a while, but she remembered Carol Brownley. Maybe because she was her own age and was so sick. She had followed up on her and she knew that Carol had improved quite a bit, but she never did pass that stone. So she was scheduled for surgery where the urologist was going to try to smash it with a laser. And the surgery was this week, if Marilou remembered correctly. Maybe she'd stop up and say hello to her while she was still in the holding area, she thought. She wanted to wish her well.

So this particular morning, Marilou was called to the I.V.P. room to inject the intravenous contrast for another kidney test. This patient was an out-patient, she knew. Picking up her tourniquet, Marilou walked into the room. There on the table was Carol Brownley. And she looked perfectly fine.

Carol started to talk to Marilou. And she talked and talked. It seemed that after the pain had subsided, Carol had been sent home. She knew that they were giving her time to pass the kidney stone, but she also knew she probably wouldn't do so. But after going through those horrible hours, Carol had decided that one way or another she was going to get that stone out of her.

A friend had told Carol that he had heard from someone else, who heard from yet another person, that there was a way to work a big stone like that down her ureter and into the bladder. He advised her to sit in a boiling hot bathtub and bear down, and to continue bearing down on and off for many hours every day. The friend told her that little by little, with the heat relaxing the smooth muscle of the ureter, that stone would move.

So for three days Carol Brownley spent most of her time in the bathtub. And she alternately pushed and then relaxed, pushed and then relaxed. And to check the progress of her labors, she inserted her finger up her vagina and pressed it up against where she guessed was the base of her bladder. After all, that's what the friend of the friend did. She was looking for that stone which she knew would eventually come down the ureter and fall into her bladder. And then, by gravity, it would fall to the bottom of the bladder, right on top of her urethra where she would feel it.

Crazy? Sure. But guess what? After three days of doing this, Carol thought she felt that kidney stone. And then she was sure of it. It was real, and she was going to get it out of her. So back to her trusty bathtub, Carol went. She sat in the hot water and pushed and pushed. And, through the wall of her vagina, she felt something hard. And that hard little thing was getting lower and lower along the front of her vagina. Didn't it hurt to do that, asked Marilou? After all, she was really picking her own kidney stone out. It hurt a little, answered Carol. But she wanted that thing out of her body, and she knew this was going to work.

Well, the morning after the second day of picking, Carol found a little pebble in her underpants. And of course, it was the kidney stone. It must have come out while she was asleep, even though she had been sure she was going to have to urinate it out along with a gigantic spasm of pain. But she didn't even have to do that. There it was.

So Carol Brownley had called her doctor who told her to come in for another I.V.P. And that was the whole story, and she was one hundred percent positive that there would be no stone in these pictures. Marilou didn't know what to say. She and Dawn, the x-ray technologist, just kept looking at each other in disbelief. How could someone pick out her own kidney stone? It couldn't happen. Could it?

Well, after the dye injection, the series of films were repeated. And there was no stone. Carol had indeed gotten rid of it. The surgery was canceled and Carol Brownley went home, after telling Marilou and Dawn, "I told you so!" When they spoke to the urologist, he told them that he had heard of this only once before and that person had worn a hole in the wall between the urethra and vagina which needed to be repaired surgically. But Carol Brownley was fine.

So that was the story -- the whole cotton pickin, rather stone pickin story. And it's true.

The Nightmare

It was two o'clock in the morning, and Christine had been a mother for just under an hour. She was in the recovery room of the maternity suite when she began to complain of chest pain. Her husband and parents were with her.

The pain hit her suddenly and she sat up straight in her bed. Christine couldn't breathe. Within minutes she was blue, her eyes back in her head.

They called a code. And as anyone who works in hospitals knows, a call for the cardiac arrest team to the obstetrical floor is a horror. It is obviously for the mother since general codes are not called for newborn babies in trouble. And obstetrical patients give life; they are not supposed to lose it.

Within two minutes, blood started to pour from Christine. It came from her vagina in streams and poured over the sides of the bed. Christine's family started to scream at what they saw, and her father fainted. The nurses tried to get them out of the unit, but they seemed to be frozen in horror. None of them could move.

Everyone worked frantically. They did everything, gave her everything. And still the blood came. It poured out in rivers, as if a bottle had been opened and turned upside down. And Christine's heart monitor stayed in a flat line. The code continued for almost an hour. Nobody wanted to stop, to admit that this girl was dead. After all, how could this happen? She was young and strong and healthy and had just given birth to a baby.

By the time the code was called, everyone was crying. The recovery area looked like a butcher shop, covered with bright fresh blood. The obstetrical nurses who had just taken care of Christine and helped deliver her healthy baby were in shock. The I.C.U. nurses, who answer all the cardiac arrest calls in the hospital, were devastated. The obstetrician, who had cared for Christine all through the happy times of her pregnancy and who had rejoiced with her when her big strong baby boy was delivered, was grief stricken. And everyone else who had worked so terribly hard to save Christine's life was in a state of shock. Should they have done an emergency hysterectomy? Would that have saved her? But how could they have done surgery? Christine was dead. She had died instantly.

How could such a joyous event become such a horrible disaster? What happened? Christine's husband ran from the unit and out of the hospital, sobbing hysterically. Her parents, when they finally left the building, were literally holding each other up.

It took quite a while for the staff to recover from this event. Christine's husband could not bring himself to take his baby home, not without his wife there. The baby was temporarily put into the custody of his grandparents.

One person very much affected was the cardiologist who had been called. He remembers being awakened from a deep sleep with the call that a brand new mother's heart had stopped, and thinking that maybe he had dreamed the whole thing. The idea was so foreign to him that he had called upstairs when he first arrived at the hospital to see if it had really happened or was just a nightmare. It was real.

The cause of death was finally determined to be an extremely rare but deadly complication of childbirth. Christine had suffered an amniotic fluid embolus, a state in which amniotic fluid is embolized into the pulmonary circulation. She had responded as though a massive blood clot had traveled to her lungs, and this tremendous insult to the body had resulted in the rapid depletion of all of her normal clotting factors. The open wound left by the separated placenta then allowed for the blood to pour out of the vascular system, and Christine rapidly bled to death.

About a month after the tragedy, the cardiologist received a call from the young husband. He still didn't understand what had happened. The doctor spent a long time on the phone, explaining this complicated and confusing process in a way that the man could somewhat comprehend. When they finally hung up, the doctor felt so much better. He realized that he, along with others, needed this chance for closure. While this nightmare would never be forgotten, it could be put to rest. Now, they could all go on.

Atlantic City

It was a drizzly afternoon in Atlantic City. Lucia had forced herself to take a break from those quarter slot machines in the casino. As usual, she was losing her money. This particular half hour had been rough, with the one armed bandits just gobbling up her coins without even letting her break even for awhile.

So Lucia had gone out on the boardwalk and had walked for a bit. The casino hotels stood together, one after the other, and they all seemed to call to her to come in and try her luck. Lucia never played the tables; in fact she never played anything higher than quarter machines. It was lucky she didn't live closer to Atlantic City, she thought. She really believed she would be dialing "1-800-GAMBLER" on a routine basis.

So Lucia, knowing it was time for a break, bought herself a cup of coffee and a gigantic chocolate chip cookie at one of those concession stands. That one cookie probably was equal to eating an entire bag all by herself, but she rationalized that with all the walking she was doing, she was most likely burning up all the fat and calories. Oh, yeah. Right. All that walking.

Well, anyway, there was Lucia with her coffee, which was much too hot to drink right away. So she walked slowly along, trying not to spill the contents of the cup all over herself. Lucia could see a crowd of people just ahead, up by the railing which separated the wooden boardwalk from the steps going down to the beach. She continued walking and saw a man lying face down on the ground. He was very still.

At first Lucia thought the guy was dead or at least unconscious, but then she noticed that there were two uniformed security guards standing over him. One had his foot on the man's back and he was talking into a walkie-talkie. The man was obviously wide awake and he lay there very still with his hands at his sides. From what she made out from the conversations around her, Lucia realized that the man had mugged someone, stolen the cup full of coins, and bolted from the casino. But he had been caught.

Good, Lucia thought. Why, that could have been me! He could have grabbed my quarters as easily as anyone else's! Just then a police car appeared, making its way slowly up the boardwalk through the crowds of people. It had driven right up the ramp from the street, Lucia realized. Oh, boy, she thought with excitement. Now I'm going to see some action. It's probably going to be just like on "Cops".

Well, the cop who got out of the car looked like he was about twelve years old. And he seemed to be totally bored with the whole scene. Moving at the speed of a snail, he bent over the man (or the "perp", as Lucia would have liked him to be called) and put handcuffs on him. Yawning out loud for a second time, the officer said in a barely audible voice, "Get up." The man stood and walked calmly with the policeman. Expressionless, he got into the back seat of the police car. The twelve year old cop, yawning once again, drove off down the boardwalk as slowly as he had arrived. How very boring, Lucia thought. She was obviously disappointed.

Lucia turned around and began to walk back the way she had come. The crowd, which seemed almost as disinterested as the policeman, had already dispersed. Within a minute or two, Lucia realized there was another group of people up ahead. And again, it was obvious that someone was lying on the ground.

So Lucia started to trot on down the boardwalk, juggling the gigantic chocolate chip cookie and the steaming cup of coffee, and thinking to herself that maybe now she would see some action. She came upon the crowd which was standing around a lady. Aside from the fact that she was lying on the ground, the lady looked perfectly fine. The woman was clutching her pocketbook, and even though she was flat on her back had her arm securely through its handle. Even the lady's makeup was perfect. She was smiling.

Within a minute or two, it became clear to Lucia that this was the lady who had been mugged by the guy who had just left in the patrol car. There was a policeman standing next to the lady, and like the first officer, he also seemed to be quite bored. At least this guy appeared to be out of his teens, Lucia thought to herself. Nobody was saying anything. People were just waiting.

Then, after what seemed like an awfully long time, an ambulance came slowly up on the boardwalk, up the same ramp that the police car had come. Two E.M.T.'s climbed out and began to ask the lady a few questions. Then they put a collar on her neck and began to roll her onto a backboard.

By this time, quite a few people had gathered and the medics had to repeatedly ask the crowd to step back so they could do what they were doing. There was an older couple blocking the way and ignoring the requests to move. The bored policeman walked over slowly and asked them if they were with the woman on the ground. Oh, no, they told the cop. They were just looking.

Lucia shook her head. It was just like at work. Lucia had been an emergency department nurse for many years, and lots of times she had seen families of her patients walking around the E.R., taking in all the sights. When she or any of the other nurses would ask these people if they needed something, they said the same thing. Oh, no.

153

They were just looking. Just as if they were in a department store or something. Browsing. What nerve, Lucia thought. Talk about being pushy!

It was just then that Lucia took a look at herself. Oh, my God, she thought. Here I am standing over this lady, coming very close to scalding her to death by dripping my burning hot coffee all over her. It was bad enough that the crumbs from the chocolate chip cookie were blowing all over the place. It would be a stroke of luck if a chunk of cookie didn't drop into her eye and give her a corneal abrasion. Or worse. Lucia started to laugh out loud. She looked like a vulture. She was actually chomping food and slurping coffee right over this poor lady's face, as if she were having refreshments while watching some form of entertainment.

And this lady wasn't even hurt. All the horrible and traumatic stuff she saw on a daily basis never even fazed her any more, but now she had become one of the group of nosey nervy privacy invaders just like the rest of this crowd. She couldn't tear herself away. Unbelievable.

Oh, well, Lucia thought. It was time to leave. The lady, by this time, was being put into the ambulance. Lucia figured she was probably fine, but needed all the medical stuff for when she decided to sue the casino or something. Lucia walked back inside through the big revolving doors. She felt very strange, kind of surprised and ashamed at the same time. She shouldn't have stayed there and become part of the crowd. She should have known better.

Lucia knew that now she was doomed to lose a couple more rolls of quarters. After all, Donald Trump needed her money, didn't he? He had gotten to depend on her routine donations to his casinos. She picked up the pace and went inside. Within fifteen minutes she had lost thirty dollars. And somehow, Lucia felt better.

154

What Time Is It?

After all these years, she couldn't even remember why he came to the hospital. But shell never forget him.

Mr. Caruso had been admitted just an hour or two before Jane arrived to work her night shift. Jane had a very large patient load, and, almost an hour into her shift, hadn't gotten to see everyone yet. So doing things the way she always did on nights like these, Jane poured her twelve o'clock meds, and made her first rounds as she passed them out. She usually did her first assessment this way, and checked out all her patients at that time. It was a good system.

It seemed as if Mr. Caruso had been ringing his bell every five minutes for that first hour of the shift, always to ask the same question. The evening staff said that he'd been doing that since the time of his admission. "What time is it?" he repeated, each time someone answered his light. Jane, continuing on her rounds, had been interrupted several times to give Mr. Caruso the time. Each time she'd answer him, he'd simply say, "O.K."

Jane was outside his door the next time that the call light came on. She stuck her head in and said, "Mr. Caruso, I'm right outside. I'll be right in." Mr. Caruso just stared at her tensely. "What time is it?" he asked again. Jane looked at her watch for what seemed like the hundredth time. "It's twelve oh four," she answered.

"Oh, good," sighed Mr. Caruso, with a little smile. "It's O.K. now." And then Mr. Caruso took a last breath and died.

Well, they called a code and worked on him for a while but it was no use. Mr. Caruso was could not be resuscitated. Something felt strange to Jane. She didn't know what it was, but it seemed to her as if Mr. Caruso had been waiting for the next day to come before he could die peacefully.

When Jane came in the following night, she told the evening nurse what had happened and how odd the whole thing had seemed. The evening nurse didn't answer for a few seconds. Then she said to Jane, "You know, the first thing he said to me when we admitted him was that his wife had Alzheimer's disease and is in a nursing home. He said that it was their forty-fifth wedding anniversary and that it wouldn't be right to leave her on their anniversary. I didn't know what he meant."

Jane and the evening nurse just looked at each other and smiled. They bot
knew, now, what Mr. Caruso had meant. O.K., Mr. Caruso, thought Jane. You mad
it. Rest well.

On The Road Again

"Mrs. Parks has to go to X-ray," Pearl called out to Corinne.

Corinne and Mary looked at each other and groaned out loud. Mrs. Parks had been in an auto accident and was recovering from multiple fractures as well as internal injuries. She had almost every tube known to mankind in her seventy year old body and she was attached to six different intravenous drips. Just that morning, Mrs. Parks had finally been weaned off the respirator and extubated, but needed a high concentration flow mask to keep her oxygen saturations within reasonable limits.

A foley catheter was in her bladder, complete with a continuous saline irrigation to wash blood clots out of her urinary system. She had a chest tube in each side, along with several abdominal sumps to drainage pumps. And to top all of this off, Mrs. Parks was in skeletal traction. She had been placed in one of those old ugly heavy steel orthopedic beds, which probably weighed thirty tons or so, not to mention the heavy weights which dangled from the traction over the foot of the bed. The doctor who wanted the nurses to bring her down to X-ray, or to anywhere, was dreaming. Actually it was more than a dream; it was a nightmare.

Corinne called out to Pearl and asked her to page whoever the brilliant physician was who had ordered the X-ray. It seemed that it was the senior resident. Dr. Berlenger answered and told them that the senior attending definitely wanted a the chest x-ray to be done down in the department, not portable. It was out of his hands, he apologized.

A half hour later, the staff was finally assembled and ready to leave for their road trip. A cardiac monitor and portable oxygen tank had been piled on the bed with Mrs. Parks, and all her infusion pumps had been consolidated onto two extra I.V. poles. The chest tube setups and all the drainage bags had been hooked to various places. All her tubes and wires (known as her plumbing equipment) were secured as well as possible, and the entourage started out.

The immovable clunker of a bed began its journey down the hall, the weights swinging wildly in the breeze and smashing noisily against the bottom of the bed frame. The bed, which was probably a thousand years old, hardly moved. The nurses were sweating up a storm before they even turned the corner. They seemed to be dragging the bed, rather than rolling it. And naturally, the I.V. poles had wheels which were almost rusted solid. It was a joke, except it wasn't exactly funny. And Mrs. Parks, he sedation having worn off at that precise minute, was howling out loud like a werewolf.

Finally, the group got the bed around the corner and past the cut-through to th next building. It was right at that point where the texture of the floor changed, jus enough to catch the wheels of one of the slowly moving I.V. poles. The pole lurched t a stop, but the momentum of the heavy bags and glass bottles didn't, and the entire pole weighed down by its green flashing infusion pumps, pitched forward. In a split secon it hit the ground, bringing the plastic bags dripping their precious liquids with it. Th bags were not the problem. It was the completely full yellow bottle o hyperalimentation fluid which shattered into two hundred thousand sticky gooey fift percent glucose coated splinters which caused a bit of trouble.

Well, needless to say, this caravan came to a halt. Someone had to run back t the I.C.U. to get another bottle of fluid and new tubing, and right then and there the had to take care of Mrs. Parks' now open central line which had the potential of suckin; air into her subclavian vein. They tried to contain the broken glass and covered th disgusting mess on the floor with wet towels. Ten minutes later, the group started u; again. When they finally reached the elevators, the nurses were cursing under thei breaths. This was unreal. Unbelievable. And they hadn't even gotten off their floor yet

By the time they got Mrs. Parks on and off the elevator, they had had it. The; were exhausted. Since it had taken so long to get to the X-ray department, the roon waiting for Mrs. Parks was now in use, and so there was a wait. The nurses didn mind. They needed to rest.

Obviously, Mrs. Parks was not going to be moved to an x-ray table. The picture; were taken with her in her own bed. This was one time they were thankful that she was in traction. The trip back upstairs, besides being backbreakingly hard, wa uneventful. That is, until they attempted to move the bed out of the elevator. And tha was when the old metal wheel on the gigantic steel bed got caught in the crack betweer the elevator car and the door. It wouldn't budge. It was jammed in there solid. The alarm in the elevator began to buzz wildly, signaling that something or someone was ir the way. And the big old door started to open and slam, open and slam, open and slam again and again against Mrs. Parks's bed. The banging and the crashing and the buzzing along with the wailing and howling of the Werewolf Parks sounded like a murder wa; being committed down in the bowels of the New York City subway system.

Try as they might, the nurses could not get that bed moving. They pushed anc they pulled and they even tried to lift the bed. It wouldn't budge. Frustrated beyond belief, Corinne ran to the first nurses station and asked for help. The nursing staff there were running up and down and around like nuts, and weren't exactly thrilled with ropping what they were doing to go work as moving men. But, since nurses help each other, they came.

The decision was that the only way to free the wheel was to lift up the entire foot f the ninety ton bed. So, with the door still crashing open and closed, and the buzzing nd the screaming still in progress, five nurses lifted straight up at the count of three. As ie bed raised off the floor, however, the jammed wheel stayed right where it was. It /as stuck solid, right there in that crack. The nurses at the back end of the elevator hoved the bed forward at that exact moment, the end result being that the bed lurched head and then slammed back down. It did so, however, minus the front left wheel.

"Oh, my God," moaned Corinne and Mary in unison. "Just go," whimpered Corinne. "Please. Just go." So go they did, on three wheels. The group pushed that ron monster down the hall. The bed moved along, traction clanging, on three wheels, he front literally being carried by three nurses. By the time they arrived back in the .C.U. they all thought they were going to pass out. At least it was over. They left Mrs. 'arks' bed looking like a big old truck with a flat tire, and went in to the chart room to it down before they fell down.

Just at that time, Dr. Berlenger walked in. "Hi, girls," he said with a broad smile. Now, don't get mad at me, but I made a little mistake. It wasn't Mrs. Parks who leeded that x-ray. It was Mrs. Conklin. Can you get her down there?"

Dr. Berlenger, to this very day, has no idea just how very close he came to being :illed at that exact moment, right there in that report room. He truly doesn't know how ucky he was that he was simply shoved out of the room and the door slammed in his ace. Nobody, absolutely nobody, except other nurses, has any concept of what these oad trips mean. And someday, somehow, the tables will turn, and these doctors will earn exactly what their few scribbled illegible words in a chart mean when they are ranslated into the world of reality.

Some how, some way, it will happen.

Ouch!

The little old lady had just been transferred in to the step down area from the coronary care unit. Unlike most patients who worry about leaving the security of the C.C.U., this lady seemed genuinely glad to be gone.

Mary Ann was getting her settled in her new bed and had just finished orienting her to the unit. "You know, dear," said Mrs. MacKenzie, "I certainly hope you girls are nicer to me than those nurses in the heart unit."

"Why, what do you mean?" asked Mary Ann, totally confused. Everybody usually raved about the care they received in the coronary care unit.

"Well, dear," explained Mrs. MacKenzie, "I was leaning over the side rail to get something out of my drawer and the next thing I knew, two nurses came running in, pushed me back into the bed and one of them punched my right in my chest! Can you imagine? And afterwards they apologized and said something about a rhythm or something. You know, dear, just because a person disturbed their routine is no reason to hit her."

Mary Ann couldn't help it. She laughed out loud. "Oh, Mrs. MacKenzie," said Mary Ann. "I think we need to have a little talk."

The Littlest Angels

As soon as she woke up, she knew it was going to be a bad day. She had been dreaming all night, dreams she couldn't remember now, but that uncomfortable sensation was there. It was what she referred to as the "doom feeling", that something bad was going to happen.

The sky matched her mood. Just yesterday it had been beautiful, a glorious late spring day with bright sunshine and a light cool breeze. Now the weather had changed drastically, and she could feel the chill in the air coming into her bedroom. The rain came down in torrents, hitting the window panes. Jill didn't want to get up to go to work. She had been off for a couple of days, and today was going to be bad. She just knew it.

Jill arrived in the I.C.U. about ten minutes late, something she never liked to do. She needed that morning cup of coffee before she started report, and now she had to hold up the night staff. When the morning rundown began, Jill learned there were three kids in their sixteen bed intensive care unit. There were no special pediatric I.C.U.'s back then; critically ill children and adults were routinely mixed together. The units did not have any individual rooms and patients were all in one big unit where they could be watched together. That setup was good for nurses, but bad for patients and their families. There was, of course, no privacy at all.

Christine was two years old. A picture of her stood on the table next to the bed. She was smiling and hugging a big brown teddy bear which was almost bigger than she was. But the real Christine, today, did not come close to what that picture showed. It seemed that yesterday, during that bright and sunny afternoon, Christine's father had accidentally rolled his car right over Christines's body. She had been in the back yard with her mother, and had toddled around front without her mom seeing her. Dad had stopped the car when he felt the bump, and when he got out to check what had happened, he saw his baby under the wheel with bright blood spurting from her mouth.

Today, Christine's body had swelled to twice its size, and was covered with bluish red blotches. The blood vessels in her skin had burst from the pressure of the car and she had bled everywhere, including into her brain. On a respirator and completely unresponsive, Christine was going to die. She had extensive brain damage.

Peter was another two year old. He had undergone surgery yesterday, an exploratory laparotomy. Full of cancer, Peter was an "open and close," which was an all too common occurrence in those days, since this was way before the breakthrough in childhood cancer treatment. Just a week earlier, before his tummy aches had started, Peter seemed to be the picture of health. The baby of four children, Peter's life expectancy was now considered to be only a few weeks.

Roberta was ten, and another statistic of the "perfect" yesterday. She had been out riding her bike and had been hit by a truck. The driver, hysterical, said he never saw her until she went flying through the air and landed on her face. Roberta had such an extensive head injury that pieces of her brain literally were sticking out through the massive areas of skull fracture. The tissue was gray, and stained with red. Gray matter. Real gray matter. The part of the brain that makes us human beings. And it was sticking out. A huge white dressing covered her head and the old fashioned Bird respirator delivered sixteen breaths per minute to her bruised lungs.

In those days, one nurse took care of the pediatric I.C.U. patients for the shift, but that morning they weren't really sure if that was the right thing to do. How could one nurse handle three dying kids? Jill was the only nurse without children of her own, so she volunteered to take all three. She could handle it, she thought, knowing now what her "doom feeling" was all about. She soon learned that it wasn't the kids who were the problem; it was the parents. The overwhelming factor was guilt. The mother who turned her back on Christine and let her wander away. The father who ran over his own precious daughter. The parents who thought Peter's belly aches were routine nothings. The mom and dad who let their ten year old girl ride her bicycle on the street. It was the worst day Jill had ever experienced since she had become a nurse.

Christine looked like a freak; she was totally unrecognizable. Her father sat at the bedside and retched and vomited continuously into a towel. Her mother, beside herself, walked in and out of the unit. She couldn't look at her child, who still had outlines of the tire treads covering the length of her body. From time to time she patted her husband on the back, and then broke out in tears. Her husband didn't seem to even know she was there.

Peter's parents sat by his bedside, saying nothing. The child, heavily sedated from the surgery, moaned occasionally, but slept most of the time. Tubes protruded from everywhere. Every so often, Peter's mom and dad looked at each other in disbelief and just shook their heads.

Roberta's mother and grandmother visited for short periods. Crying continuously, they tried to speak to her around their tears, hoping against hope that she could hear them. At one point, Roberta's twelve year old sister came to the door to ask if she could visit. Jill, knowing that Roberta's basketball sized head with its distorted unrecognizable face would be the way the child would always remember her sister,

162

imply told her no. Whether that was right or wrong, it was what Jill decided. Roberta was too sick for visitors, Jill told her.

The day was a nightmare. Nobody really knows how the staff made it through the shift. Just before it ended, Jill saw Dr. Collus, the chief resident in surgery, go up to Roberta's bed. Her family was not there. He stood there a while, looking at the child. Then turning to Jill, he said softly, "This kid is dead. She just doesn't know it yet." And with that he pulled the hose attached to the Bird respirator off the end of the endotracheal tube and threw it down on the floor. With tears streaming down his cheeks, Dr. Collus turned and left the unit. Dr. Collus had ten year old twin girls of his own.

Jill gave report and left the hospital. The staff purposely waited until she was gone before they told Roberta's family that her heart had stopped. Jill drove home in silence, a sick feeling in the pit of her stomach. When she got home she went into the bathroom and threw up, and then she began to cry.

Two days later, Christine died. Her parents, unable to look at her any more, were not at the hospital. Peter was transferred to the pediatric ward where he lived for another three weeks. He died during the night in the arms of his father.

Maybe some day we will all understand the reason why tragedies like these happen. Most probably, we will not. Meanwhile, life goes on and as sure as it does, more horrible things will happen to innocent little children. And all we can do is believe that they are the little angels lent to us here on earth for a very special purpose, as a gift to be treasured for the time they are ours.

163

Epilogue

"She used to be a nurse."

Nobody "used to be a nurse." Nurses are nurses forever. Just because someone ; not officially practicing does not mean she has given up nursing. That can't be done.

The profession of nursing is so unique that it can't be compared to anything else. he caring, the compassion, and the emotional commitment becomes part of the person. hat's what nursing is all about.

There are many reasons why nurses leave the health care environment. Family esponsibility, health problems, even what we call "burnout" all are factors. But what nade us choose nursing in the first place stays forever.

I've been a nurse for more years than I care to mention. And I know I still can do , and do it well. But when the time comes and I have to leave, I'll still be a nurse. It's vhat I am.

Today I was cleaning out some old papers in a drawer and came across some etters from some families of patients I took care of a very long time ago. Some of the vords will stay with me when things get tough. "Neither words nor flowers could ossibly express our appreciation for the hours of love and affection that you so aithfully gave," one card read. Another said, "God could scarcely know the good that le created when he persuaded you to become a nurse." And another said, "I shall lways be grateful that it was you who was Phillip's nurse that last day and that you vere with him when he died." And still another said, "If only you could know how nuch you helped. By just being there, you gave me tremendous comfort."

And there are more.

Sometimes, when we get caught up in the tasks we have to do and when we omplain about the overwork and understaffing, we forget for a while what it means to »e a nurse. We all need to give ourselves a little space, a little time, to try to remember vhy we became nurses in the first place. The old saying, "Take time along the way to mell the flowers," rings true. We are privileged to be part of the joy and of the sadness of so many lives.

Did you ever go to pay your respects at a patient's wake or even stop by a nemorial service of a particularly special patient? Did you notice the faces of the amily members when they saw you? "Look, it's Bill's nurse!" they say to their relatives,

164

as they proudly bring you around to meet people. "She took such good care of Bill"
they announce. You have, for that short time, become a beloved member of the family.

Look at the bulletin boards and walls of any nurses' station, clinic, or office. It's
full of letters of praise and thanks. And did you ever wonder why it's so hard for nurses
to lose weight? Just take a look at the tables and desks of any nursing unit. They're
filled with cakes and cookies and candy from grateful families!

A nurse, no matter where she works, is like nobody else. She works harder,
moves faster, and accomplishes more than anyone else. Nurses care about each other,
and no matter how tired they are, they always give their all. To their patients and to
each other.

The reason that a nurse always remains a nurse is obvious. Nursing is such a
unique profession that people know right away if they can make it. And if they can't,
they leave it right at the beginning. So anyone who becomes a nurse can never do
anything else. To be a nurse is to join a family. Certainly, we aren't perfect and there
are times when things are not ideal, but that's what happens in any family.

A nurse does anything and everything. She can cope. He can handle the
unexpected, because the unexpected is always expected. That's what happens when
you become part of someone else's life. A nurse is a nurse forever. Oh, maybe the
nurse is away from the hospital or school or clinic or wherever she used to work, but the
nurse part of the person stays.

I'd like to paraphrase something I read many years ago when I was a student at
New York's Mount Sinai Hospital:

> *Surely, someday up in heaven there will be a special*
> *group of God's angels running around dressed in*
> *white uniforms or colored scrubs or even street clothes.*
> *They will be wearing stethoscopes around their necks*
> *instead of halos around their heads, and they will be*
> *carrying medication trays with big doses of T.L.C., instead*
> *of harps. And everyone will know that back on Earth, these*
> *angels used to be the very special group of people . . . .*
>
> **known as nurses.**